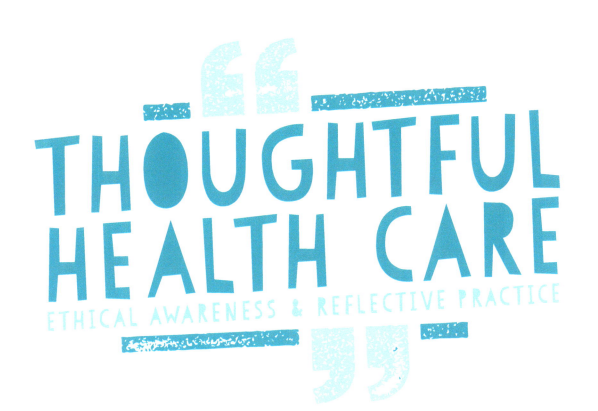

Sara Miller McCune founded SAGE Publishing in 1965 to support the dissemination of usable knowledge and educate a global community. SAGE publishes more than 1000 journals and over 800 new books each year, spanning a wide range of subject areas. Our growing selection of library products includes archives, data, case studies and video. SAGE remains majority owned by our founder and after her lifetime will become owned by a charitable trust that secures the company's continued independence.

Los Angeles | London | New Delhi | Singapore | Washington DC | Melbourne

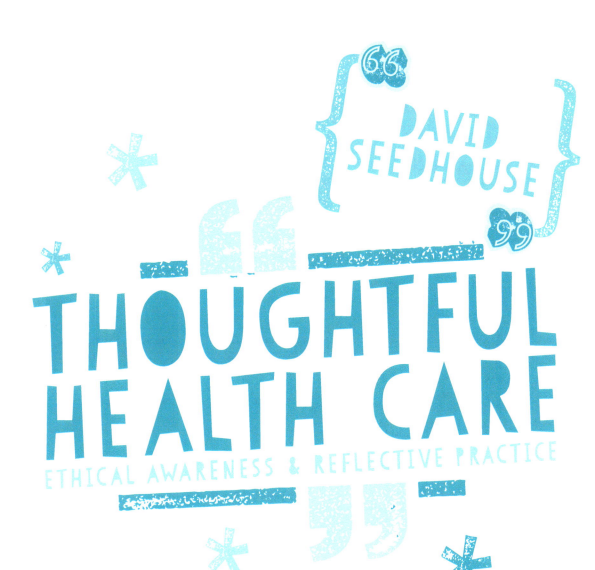
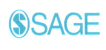

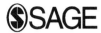

Los Angeles | London | New Delhi
Singapore | Washington DC | Melbourne

SAGE Publications Ltd
1 Oliver's Yard
55 City Road
London EC1Y 1SP

SAGE Publications Inc.
2455 Teller Road
Thousand Oaks, California 91320

SAGE Publications India Pvt Ltd
B 1/I 1 Mohan Cooperative Industrial Area
Mathura Road
New Delhi 110 044

SAGE Publications Asia-Pacific Pte Ltd
3 Church Street
#10-04 Samsung Hub
Singapore 049483

Editor: Becky Taylor
Assistant editor: Charlène Burin
Production editor: Katie Forsythe
Copyeditor: Bryan Campbell
Indexer: Adam Pozner
Marketing manager: Tamara Navaratnam
Cover design: Wendy Scott
Typeset by: C&M Digitals (P) Ltd, Chennai, India
Printed and bound by CPI Group (UK) Ltd,
Croydon, CR0 4YY

© David Seedhouse 2017

First published 2017

Apart from any fair dealing for the purposes of research or private study, or criticism or review, as permitted under the Copyright, Designs and Patents Act, 1988, this publication may be reproduced, stored or transmitted in any form, or by any means, only with the prior permission in writing of the publishers, or in the case of reprographic reproduction, in accordance with the terms of licences issued by the Copyright Licensing Agency. Enquiries concerning reproduction outside those terms should be sent to the publishers.

Library of Congress Control Number: 2016956254

British Library Cataloguing in Publication data

A catalogue record for this book is available from the British Library

ISBN 978-1-4739-5382-6
ISBN 978-1-4739-5383-3 (pbk)

At SAGE we take sustainability seriously. Most of our products are printed in the UK using FSC papers and boards. When we print overseas we ensure sustainable papers are used as measured by the PREPS grading system. We undertake an annual audit to monitor our sustainability.

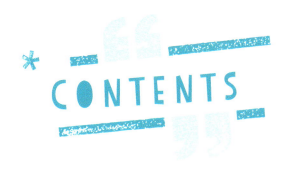

About the Author	*vi*
Acknowledgements	*vii*
Publisher's Acknowledgements	*viii*
Praise for the book	*ix*
Introduction: The Goblin in the Meadow	*xi*
1 The Values Delusion	1
2 Labels	32
3 Creating Reality	50
4 Odyssey	65
5 Purpose	101
6 Ethics is Everywhere	115
7 The Delusion Detector	129
8 The Toolkit	146
References	*184*
Index	*195*

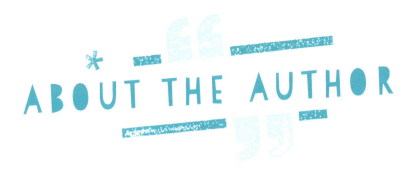

ABOUT THE AUTHOR

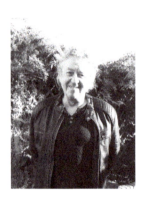

David Seedhouse is a widely-read writer on the philosophy of health care. He has written or edited 15 books, including the best-selling *Health: The Foundations for Achievement* and *Ethics: The Heart of Health Care*. David is a Visiting Professor at the University of Derby, UK, and Western Sydney University in Australia. David is also the creator of the Values Exchange – an online community for reflection and debate about ethical and social issues, used in many universities internationally, and also by the NHS in the UK. A version of the Values Exchange is connected to this book, and all readers are encouraged to sign in and enjoy the creative conversations.

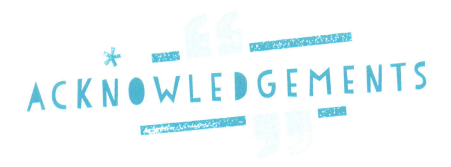

ACKNOWLEDGEMENTS

This book has emerged out of a tumultuous two years of working and personal life. I have not had the luxury of a sabbatical from university or business, or any other part of a very busy existence, so the book is no doubt less well researched than it could be – but it is the very real product of a very real life.

As usual, I don't have anyone else to blame for its errors and omissions, but I do have to thank my colleagues at Sage Publishing for their very professional support and encouragement, and for their willingness to trial the Values Exchange (my business) as an online adjunct to their textbooks. I am also deeply grateful to Vanessa Peutherer for her belief in me as a writer and human being, and for her considerable part in the creation of *Thoughtful Health Care*. Almost all the examples in the book are hers, and they lend it a reality and practical depth that I would not otherwise have been able to achieve.

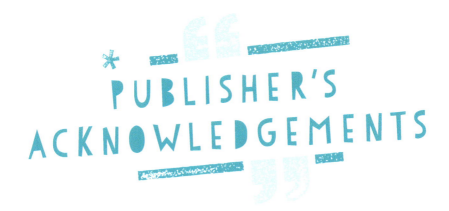

The publishers would like to thank the following individuals for their invaluable feedback on the proposal and chapters of the book:

Dr Silvana Bettiol, University of Tasmania, Australia

Dianne Burns, University of Manchester, UK

Benny Goodman, Plymouth University, UK

Angela Hudson, University of the West of England, UK

Gillian Rowe, Plymouth University Partnerships, UK

Nick Wrycraft, Anglia Ruskin University, UK

Wendy Wright, University of the West of Scotland, UK

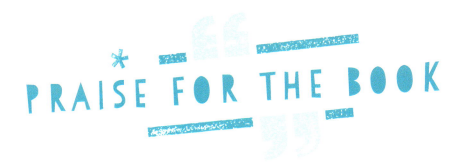

PRAISE FOR THE BOOK

Though my discipline is not health care but risk management, the writings of David Seedhouse have enlightened my thinking and influenced my worldview in invaluable ways. A practical approach underpinned by a coherent philosophy is what we need, and David delivers yet again in this latest work.

Professor David Ball, Middlesex University, UK

David Seedhouse has produced a strikingly honest view of where health policy makers have gone wrong but more importantly suggests an approach and ways health care professionals of the future can improve the quality of care for patients This is an interesting book that I was keen to read and didn't disappoint. David Seedhouse provides some challenging ideas that will make readers reflect on and question their assumptions. This is a must purchase book for undergraduate nurses.

As a trainee nurse in the optimistic 90s we were encouraged to challenge practice and question ideas. In the decades that followed we were then told to blindly follow targets regardless of the reasons for them. Currently the NHS is in crisis and badly needs leaders. David Seedhouse's excellent book reignites that spirit of curiosity and sets the challenge for health care practitioners to really look at what is health and how in moving forward do we best provide a services that delivers the best health care.

Nick Wrycraft, Anglia Ruskin University, UK

David Seedhouse is a well-known and respected author in this field and in this book delivers a corrective to the current well-meaning but erroneous views on such things as values based recruitment and the 6Cs. Any health care worker thinking critically and wanting to articulate why certain practices and values are not up to the mark would do very well in reading this. The writing style is very accessible without dumbing down. Key ideas are illustrated and examined through very appropriate case studies and think stops. This should be core reading in any nursing programme.

Benny Goodman, Plymouth University, UK

An excellent book from a trusted author. This is a really useful source of information for nurses and student nurses which encourages much discussion and debate. The writing style is engaging and the reader certainly engages in the thought provoking toolkit and practical examples.

Wendy Wright, University of the West of Scotland, UK

This critically insightful and seriously thought provoking text challenges readers to critically reflect upon and carefully consider 'the values delusion' within contemporary health care settings. Pulling no punches, Seedhouse presents a refreshing and sometimes scathing attack on some of the superficial ways in which 'values' are viewed across many sectors.

Dianne Burns, University of Manchester, UK

This thought provoking book contests the ideas of values and ethical awareness that are inherent in health and social care settings today. The reader is encouraged to reflect on established perspectives and reframe views. It is very accessible and broad in its appeal. I would recommend to all health and social care professionals.

Angela Hudson, University of the West of England, UK

When every organisation – from the NHS to CocaCola – has its list of platitudinous 'core values', on which all its practices are allegedly 'based', Seedhouse's penetrating scepticism is not only refreshing but urgently needed. This book is wilfully contentious – for the most part legitimately so. Seedhouse cares less about convincing us he is right on any given issue, much more about encouraging the genuine, critical thinking and practice that organisations agree, in principle, we need, but which so many of their structures inhibit.

Michael Loughlin, Manchester Metropolitan University, UK

INTRODUCTION
THE GOBLIN IN THE MEADOW

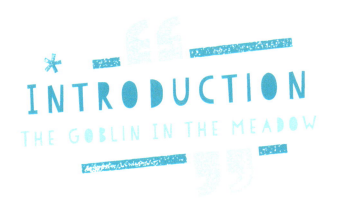

Iggy's a two-year-old black labrador. He's a knowing dog, highly attuned to his environment. When he's outside, his face twitches incessantly. His whole body's alert. His eyes see the world differently from ours. He hears and smells more than we do. He has no words to describe his experience – he just experiences.

Iggy's standing in a meadow in high summer, taking it all in: tall grasses, poppies nodding, butterflies, swooping birds, nature's quiet sounds, woodland behind – and above that, blue sky, drifting clouds, a gentle breeze and all of it swaying in some mysterious harmony. An amazing landscape. Full of colour, possibility, unknown paths, new adventures.

Then a rat hurtles from a burrow and darts past. Iggy's transfixed. The amazing landscape vanishes – only the rat exists for Iggy now. He chases it madly but the rat escapes into a bolthole. Iggy barks fiercely. Tries furiously to dig his way in. Waits. Barks some more. The rat's gone. Iggy turns away. After all there are bees in the meadow. And wasps. And endless other mysteries. There's a whole unknown world waiting in the meadow.

Now there are people in the meadow. Happy people at first. But look. Coming out of the undergrowth. It's a goblin, a scary goblin. The humans are transfixed for a split second. The amazing landscape vanishes – only the goblin exists now. The people chase it madly but the goblin escapes into a bolthole. They shout fiercely. Then they turn away – they're going to get weapons. They tell everyone they know about the goblin. They come back to the meadow and watch for it. Soon enough they fence the meadow off. Put signs up. Beware of the goblin. Go back. Danger. And the amazing landscape stays vanished. It's where the goblin lives. That's all that matters now.

The central theme of this book – you might even say the only theme – is that like Iggy, we humans should always be aware of the whole meadow, not just the part where crowds of us have gathered (1).

This book was originally intended to be an introduction to values-based health care for students and professionals. Good values are increasingly seen as essential to best practice, so a book explaining exactly what they are and how they can be effectively applied seemed an obviously good idea. Not only that, but a decade earlier I had written a scholarly textbook about values-based decision making for the caring professions, and built a website for reflective practice called the Values Exchange. It seemed a perfect fit.

Yet the more I thought about values the more it became apparent that our current understanding of them is inadequate.

There is a widely-held view that values are solid, meaningful, stable attitudes. On this view a 'compassionate person' will have the same characteristics as another 'compassionate person', will behave with 'compassion' in all circumstances, and will have associated values – like 'honesty' and 'respect' – which fit snugly with her 'compassion'. Understood like this, values can be defined in a simple way, can be readily detected from what people say and do, can be taught, and can be listed in mission statements to inspire consistent behaviours.

This reading of values has become so popular that the NHS bases its entire Constitution on its own set of values; almost all institutions and businesses proudly declare their values on their websites and office walls; students and practitioners are taught or persuaded to adopt certain values and not others; and prospective health professionals have their values assessed at interview – and may even be denied work if these values are found wanting.

Envisaged this way, values are like simple commands on memory sticks. Insert a memory stick containing the code for 'integrity' into a person's brain and *voila* – she's programmed to act 'with integrity' in every circumstance.

Trouble is, as soon as you examine real-life situations, this cosy understanding of values disintegrates. Values do inform our decisions to an extent, but in a much more vague and erratic fashion than we assume. 'Compassion', for example, might have one meaning to one person and a conflicting meaning to another. To Samantha 'compassion' might be the ability to empathise, to Benjamin 'compassion' may mean acting against a patient's wishes in their best interests. To Jules it might be 'compassionate' to assist a terminally ill person to end their life, to Andy it may be 'compassionate' to do everything he can to prevent the dying patient committing suicide: legitimate versions of 'compassion', leading to totally opposite actions.

How can a memory stick be programmed for 'compassion' if 'compassion' can inform logically incompatible choices?

Not only that, but there is massive evidence – both from academic research and everyday life – that we are much more inconsistent in our choices and actions than we like to think. Dependent on what's happening in our daily lives, our emotional state, our level of knowledge, who we are friendly with, who we are working with, how busy we are, how stressed we are and so on, we may one day act according to one version of 'compassion', and contradict it the next.

The Official View is that values are fundamental drivers of our behaviours, but with just a little reflection it's obvious that our choices are formed by more powerful forces: by our peers, friends and colleagues, by our biology, by our psychology (and its errors), by our personalities, by our cultures, by our personal histories, by our education, by our environment and countless other factors.

How can the Official View be so at odds with what every thoughtful person knows from normal life experience? How can so many apparently intelligent people be so wrong about the nature of values? What is it that's blinding us to the depth of people's thought processes, loyalties and decision making? Why do so many of us need to simplify the richness of life by substituting myths for reality?

The more I thought about it the more I saw the Official View of values as a form of delusion – once you look at it closely, it's hard to think of it as anything else. Then I wondered, is this delusion unique to health care or is it everywhere in human life? What does the delusion consist of, what are its implications, how in particular does it impact on health care and – most important of all – can we escape it? Can we become more aware of ourselves, more conscious of the perplexing nature of life, and more accepting of inconsistency if that is the way things really are? If we can see past at least some of our delusion, will it enable us to be more sensitive and helpful to other people?

These are big questions, but I hope this book goes at least a little way toward answering them. It begins in a straightforward fashion, examining the way values are understood in health care, and showing by analysis and example that this understanding is mistaken – in fact it's almost completely wrong. Then, in an attempt to get closer to the bottom of things, we embark on an unusual – but I hope entertaining – investigation into a range of social phenomena: from risk, schools, rights and progress to the news-media and even the survival strategies of plants.

We are driven to make sense of the world. In order to do so we stick as many labels on it as we can, but the more complex and ingrained our labelling systems become the more we lose sight of everything we haven't or can't label. We believe our labels are true, and we are all too easily convinced that the rules and policies we make up would somehow exist even if we didn't.

Worse still, our labels make it appear as if the world is made up of separate parts or packets, when really everything is profoundly connected.

Our worst delusion is to imagine that we can improve the social world by trying to change it as we see and define it, rather than work with its astonishing intricacies, as best we can. Things are just not as simple as they seem.

Thoughtful Health Care offers a Toolkit for thoughtful practice in complex reality. Though it's easier to offer catchy lists of key words and simplistic appeals to 'put patients first' – if reality is more complicated than we like to think it is, trying to change it as if it's straightforward is just not going to work. Accordingly, the Toolkit is rich and varied, and requires intelligence and perception to use. It's more a compendium of insights than a set of spanners, but it's surely less deluded than the official alternatives. With effort and practice the Toolkit offers much-needed support for health workers and students currently overwhelmed and frustrated by disconnected codes, missions, rules and checklists.

Overall, *Thoughtful Health Care* offers a timely reminder that there's so much more to working life than obediently following the latest rules and policies. All health workers have a rich blend of knowledge, experience and intuition. They work with other complex people, most of whom have temporary or permanent vulnerabilities – creating an unpredictable mix of action and reaction. While rules and codes and disciplinary reviews may help promote consistency of care to a small extent, these highly specific labels frequently undermine creativity, curiosity, kindness and – ultimately – the capacity to respond to each person as a unique individual.

Each of my earlier books, one way or another, was designed to help health workers think more systematically about their work and purposes. These texts were meant to be accessible to any reader, yet flicking through their pages I can see why some of my work has been misunderstood, and why parts of it might turn off readers who prefer quick fixes and certainties over philosophical rigour. Though they may be clear enough to the initiated, they do contain a fair bit of technical detail, which I have left out of *Thoughtful Health Care*. However, if you are sufficiently keen to want the theoretical arguments which underpin the present book, I recommend *Health: The Foundations for Achievement*; *Ethics: The Heart of Health Care*; and *Health Promotion: Philosophy, Prejudice and Practice* (2, 3, 4). If not, just enjoy the book you have in your hands at the moment.

In *Thoughtful Health Care*, I have tried to write a different sort of book, in a different style from my more scholarly essays. Here, I simply aim to empower any interested reader with the sense that if something looks or feels dodgy it very probably is. Whenever this applies to you, the book will give you food for contemplation, and a few techniques that will help you question incongruity, even if only to satisfy yourself.

Thoughtful Health Care is meant to be a pleasant, absorbing read, with a variety of examples drawn from many areas of life, not just health care. It's intended to be treasured (ideally) – a reflective retreat for when you're overwhelmed with rules for rules' sake; or perhaps working in unintelligent systems with people who don't seem to care as much as you do. Or maybe when you have to deal with dumb unkindness, and it's damaging you, not to say others.

I have in mind a reader who would relish a quiet, thoughtful conversation with a moderately educated, unafraid man – perhaps shutting his or her door after a dispiriting day, sipping a coffee or a gin, and thinking quietly, 'At least I'm not alone in my thoughts and concerns. Despite the fact that I'm part of a very small minority, I'm not entirely wrong. I have a point, whatever they say.'

Thoughtful Health Care does not abandon logic or robust reasoning; it just doesn't make a meal of it. Even Chapter 1 – which is the most scathing about the latest absurdities amok in the NHS – is meant as a humourous journey. Thoughtless attempts – however well-meaning – to improve the world with codes, 'values-based recruitment', and lists of words all beginning with the same letter, are merely the over-confident assertions of people out of their intellectual depth. Seemingly all the reason in the world won't help them see this, so I suggest you stand back with a wry smile while doing all you can to make a difference, on your own terms, according to your own sense of integrity and moral commitment.

While *Thoughtful Health Care* draws on parts of my previous work, it does have something new to offer. It points to a constant choice we all have: you can look at the world as if it's an uncertain, mostly mysterious place where you learn continually, or you can look at it as if everything they tell you is true. I know which I prefer, and if you feel the same you will find much support in its pages.

This is a very personal book, which is pretty much forbidden territory in academia. But then every book, and every piece of research for that matter, is personal, however much it's disguised. So why pretend otherwise?

I've written *Thoughtful Health Care* primarily in order to communicate. And by far the most important part of any human communication is communicating yourself to others. Just as everything else in the world is inseparably connected, the author is never separate from what he writes. Nor is he separate from his readers, each of whom creates a unique reading experience as they blend their worlds with the words on a book's pages.

David Seedhouse
Wolverley, England

(Note: This book uses a dedicated Values Exchange: http://thoughtful.vxcommunity.com. The Values Exchange is a set of educational tools designed to promote self-awareness, awareness of others and to develop skills in critical thinking. It is also an extensive online learning community, which every reader of this book is invited to join.

Issues to reinforce the book's themes, to challenge the reader, and to build the community are peppered throughout the book. Simply sign in as instructed then respond to as many issues as you like.)

1 THE VALUES DELUSION

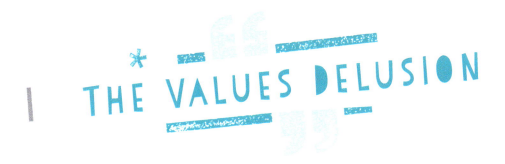

The Official View of Values

There's a widely accepted view of values, shared across many sectors of society, which goes something like this.

1. Values can be clearly differentiated from each other.
2. Values can be held and exhibited both by individuals and organisations.
3. Values can be clearly identified as consistent drivers of individual and organisational behaviours.
4. Values expressed as single words are understood in the same way by everyone who reads or hears them.
5. Lists of different values – often known as 'values statements' – can consistently guide the actions of individuals and organisations.
6. People can and should be recruited according to their values.
7. If an organisation professes the right values, it will make the right decisions.
8. Lists of values help us tell the difference between right and wrong.

This way of thinking of values is so commonplace, at first it's hard to see anything wrong with it. Yet it's mistaken in every respect, as careful inspection of any official values statement will reveal (5). For example, take the NHS Constitution, which offers the authorised list of 'principles and values that guide the NHS' (6).

According to **Principle 1**:

> **The NHS provides a comprehensive service available to all**
>
> This principle applies irrespective of gender, race, disability, age, sexual orientation, religion, belief, gender reassignment, pregnancy

and maternity or marital or civil partnership status. The service is designed to diagnose, treat and improve both physical and mental health. It has a duty to each and every individual that it serves and must respect their human rights. At the same time, it has a wider social duty to promote equality through the services it provides and to pay particular attention to groups or sections of society where improvements in health and life expectancy are not keeping pace with the rest of the population.

Several words in this paragraph are 'Big Values' words: 'duty', 'respect', 'human rights', and 'equality'. Together they seem to make an impressive point. Yet when you think about it, Principle 1 doesn't actually make sense.

The principle says the NHS will treat everyone equally and respect their human rights. It also says it will pay more attention to the most disadvantaged sectors of society, since the NHS has a duty to help the least well-off people. However, if you have limited resources (which is always the case in the NHS) and you want to give a greater proportion of these to the least advantaged people, you can't offer the same service to everyone equally, so you can't respect everyone's rights in the same way. It's like saying, here's an apple pie: everyone in our society has an equal right to the same size piece. However, the people in Poortown are thinner than everyone else so – in the interests of equality – it's only fair to make the better off people's slices smaller, in order to give more to the thin people.

You can't have it both ways. You can't say everyone has the right to the same size slice of pie and at the same time say that some people have a right to a bigger slice, when there's only so much pie to go around. There's a gigantic clash of values in Principle 1, which its authors somehow failed to notice: 'equal rights and treating everyone identically' versus 'unequal rights and treating people differently'.

It's quite an achievement to generate a deep-seated philosophical conundrum in the first paragraph of an official declaration. But while this might be a useful discussion point for a university seminar, it's entirely unhelpful in health service practice. If I'm an NHS manager responsible for distributing resources in line with NHS 'principles and values', and I want to use Principle 1 to guide me, I'm stuck in an impossible bind. Do I give everyone an equal slice of the pie or don't I?

What I think the NHS should be saying in Principle 1 is that it wants to create a more equal society, and will therefore offer more to the neediest people to try to bring them closer to the better off people – which means that the rights of better off people will sometimes have to be overridden. This does make sense and could, with much more detail, be applied in practice. However, as it stands, Principle 1 flatly contradicts one of the tenets of 'the Official View':

> **Official View 5.** Lists of different values – often known as 'values statements' – can consistently guide the actions of individuals and organisations.

Generally speaking, in addition to their vagueness of meaning, lists of values exhibit three related types of problem – theoretical, practical and ethical. Theoretical problems occur when, as with Principle 1, the itemised words and claims are incompatible in the abstract, and therefore could never be used to guide practice. Practical problems arise when the theory hangs together, but where what is claimed is happening isn't actually happening. And ethical problems happen when controversial outlooks are put forward as if everyone is bound to agree with them.

Principle 4 in the Constitution exemplifies all three types of problem:

> **The NHS aspires to put patients at the heart of everything it does**
>
> It should support individuals to promote and manage their own health. NHS services must reflect, and should be coordinated around and tailored to, the needs and preferences of patients, their families and their carers. Patients, with their families and carers where appropriate, will be involved in and consulted on all decisions about their care and treatment. The NHS will actively encourage feedback from the public, patients and staff, welcome it and use it to improve its services.

To say that NHS services must reflect the needs and preferences of patients, their families and their carers is a very big claim. Of course, it sounds perfectly reasonable at a glance, but to deliver on it consistently, *all* the needs and preferences of *all* patients and families must be met. However, in our complex social environment this simply cannot be so. There are countless examples where meeting the needs and preferences of one patient will prevent or even act against meeting the needs and preferences of another – this is just the way things are: not allowing smokers to smoke in hospital grounds, preventing windows opening to stop injury while reducing ventilation, banning flowers on wards in case of allergies, prohibiting clinicians sitting on patients' beds to reduce infection while limiting human contact, giving everyone breakfast at the same time regardless of when they usually eat, refusing to operate on one needy patient in favour of another needy patient who would benefit more – all these are examples of inevitable conflict between needs. And everyone knows that the needs and preferences of patients, families and carers are very often at odds: patients want one thing and their families want another, carers recommend a treatment and the patient doesn't want it. What is a need to one person can be a burden to another.

How, in the case below, can you – or anyone else working in the health service – possibly meet the needs and preferences of all patients, each member of their family and their carers, in a fair and equal manner?

STOP & THINK ONE: THE CURRY CONUNDRUM

Ahmed, a 65-year-old married man, is a voluntary in-patient in the Acute Mental Health Unit. He has been admitted for assessment and treatment of severe depression. Ahmed moved to England from southern India 20 years ago with his family. On admission, Ahmed is found to be underweight and he reports a moderate loss of appetite (anorexia) which has increased during his stay on the Unit and been present since his depressive symptoms have worsened. During his stay on the ward, on open questioning, it is established that Ahmed enjoys eating his wife's homemade curry but dislikes hospital food on the whole, which seems to have contributed to a steady, continual loss of weight.

You are the health worker on duty. You have spoken to Ahmed and encouraged him to fill in his daily menu choice, to allow him to choose what he would like to eat. Ahmed continues to be unmotivated and seems disinterested, but fills the form in anyway. He has also been referred to the dietician for advice by the Registered Nurse on duty.

At meal time, that evening, you notice that, as usual, Ahmed has not eaten any of the food which has arrived from the kitchens, and despite encouragement, asks you to take his tray away, with his food untouched. You report this to the nurse in charge and document your evaluation in Ahmed's notes.

At visiting time you are surprised to notice that Ahmed is sat with his wife and is visibly eating curry and rice with his hands, in front of everyone, in the day room. Some of the staff and patients verbalise feeling uncomfortable as a result of this behaviour, saying it is 'unhygienic' and 'repulsive'. These statements are made, despite the fact that Ahmed, as part of his culture, sees nothing wrong with eating his curry with his hands: as he says, 'it tastes better' and his family regularly eat in this way at home, as do well over 1 billion people around the world.

It is evident that Ahmed's wife has snuck food in for him, against the hospital policy, which states that due to legal obligations, to comply with the Food Safety Act 1990 and associated legislation and the risks of food poisoning, relatives and patients are unable to bring in meals containing cooked meat as they may support the growth of pathogenic bacteria.

What would you do in this scenario?

Do you agree with the proposal below?

It is proposed that you continue to allow Ahmed to consume his wife's curry with his hands, in the communal area.

Add your response on the Values Exchange: http://thoughtful.vxcommunity.com/Issue/think-stop-one-curry-conundrum/23053

(Case originally posted by Vanessa Peutherer, VX Learning Facilitator)

One of the main ethical problems with simplistic values statements is the repeated attempt to use them to deliver Official View 8:

> **Official View 8.** Lists of values help us tell the difference between right and wrong.

For example, the first sentence of Principle 4 is written as if it's obviously right:

> [The NHS] should support individuals to promote and manage their own health.

But why should the NHS 'support individuals to promote and manage their own health'? Why shouldn't the NHS look after people unconditionally – whether or not they want to manage their own health?

If I'm living in a damp flat, badly educated and unemployed, over fifty with few prospects, and I decide to smoke cigarettes to make myself feel better, am I a bad person for not 'promoting and managing' my own health? Maybe I am promoting my health by smoking, since it helps me cope and makes me happy? Since 'health' is not defined in the NHS Constitution, it's not clear.

Have I failed in my ethical duty to promote my own health if I'm miserable, lost and getting by in an 'unhealthy' way? Or does the NHS Constitution place unreasonable expectations on me in a situation where few of my circumstances are of my own making? Where does this value judgement – that people ought to manage their own health – come from, and how is it justified? It's certainly not a neutral position, and it definitely requires defending.

All the other principles have theoretical, practical and ethical difficulties too. They are bound to because they're grandiose and removed from the messy reality we all have to live in.

Consider other principles.

> **Access to NHS services is based on clinical need, not an individual's ability to pay**

Actual practice is much more complicated than this. For example, some health authorities will fund certain treatments while others will not, even in identical circumstances (7, 8). It's also common for patients to be seen within the NHS by part-salaried doctors, and then offered speedier private treatment by the same doctors. Not NHS treatment, admittedly, but it is 'paid for' treatment made accessible by the use of the NHS.

> **Public funds for healthcare will be devoted solely to the benefit of the people that the NHS serves**

This is plainly untrue. According to newspaper reports, in 2015 the NHS faced a potentially massive £15 billion bill for clinical negligence (9), most of which will go out either in payments to a handful of patients negligently harmed, or to law firms.

Less exorbitantly, the Report and Accounts of the NHS Litigation Authority in 2014–15 says:

> Last year we paid over £1.1 billion to patients who suffered harm and their legal representatives, this coming year it will be c £1.4 billion and with accumulated provisions in our balance sheet of over £28 billion further significant increases are already in the pipeline. Currently over a third of what we spend each year is received by the legal profession and … most of this is paid to claimants' lawyers. (10)

Vast sums of money are spent on pharmaceutical products of dubious benefit, or which actually cause harm – for example, Tardive Dyskinesia, a movement disorder, is actually caused by neuroleptic or antipsychotic drugs; and 'superbugs' which become immune to anti-biotics are increasingly alarming public health authorities (11, 12, 13, 14, 15).

Clearly it is just false to say that public funds are spent only on the public in the NHS. So why say it?

> **The NHS is accountable to the public, communities and patients that it serves**

Sadly, this is only partly true. Patients' experience of trying to redress wrongs against them, or even to get apologies for poor care, is consistently of stress, closed doors and failure (16). As a matter of fact, accountability does not always exist.

Lots More Values

The NHS Constitution is by no means the only set of values statements offered by the NHS. In addition to the Constitution, there's a further (and rather similar) iteration of supposed NHS Core Values (17); there's a strangely popular list which uses six words, all of which – ridiculously – begin with the letter C; different arms of the NHS (mental health care and health promotion, for example) each have their own set of values (18); and most NHS Trusts, not content with the general NHS Constitution, have come up with their own values schemes as well (19).

Unsurprisingly, not only does each different 'values statement' exhibit a host of theoretical, practical and ethical problems but – if you can be bothered to lump them all together – you'll see that sooner or later they end up contradicting each other.

The 6Cs

'The 6Cs' is the shallowest effort at an NHS values list so far. In November 2013, the Chief Nursing Officer, Jane Cummings, tried to explain it:

> The values that underpin our professional care have never been more important than at the present time. The Francis Report, the Keogh Report, the Cavendish and Berwick Reviews have all highlighted how we need to improve and in doing so have emphasised the centrality of compassion in the care we deliver …

She and her colleague, Viv Bennett, created a strategy, which they called 'Compassion in Practice'. The pair decided to find other positive words beginning with C to go with 'compassion', rather like trying to find curtains and lampshades to go with new wallpaper:

> … core values and behaviours recognised by patients and carers alike and which are encapsulated in the 6Cs: Care, Compassion, Competence, Communication, Courage and Commitment. Each of these key concepts has been defined through extensive consultation with patients, nurses, midwives and care staff as part of our process of engagement with the professions.

But – as we will shortly see in detail – you don't define values in consultation: values are continually exhibited by living beings, in every behaviour. To say that 'values … have never been more important than at the present time' is as irrelevant as saying 'oxygen has never been more important than at the present time': just as oxygen is essential to life, values are an essential part of our decision making. And, like us, values are complex, often vague, sometimes contradictory, and are only one part of what drives our decisions and actions.

Every one of Cummings' 6Cs is too vaguely expressed to be taken seriously. On compassion, for instance, she says:

> Compassion: is how care is given through relationships based on empathy, respect and dignity – it can also be described as intelligent kindness, and is central to how people perceive their care. (20, 21)

Pretty much every item of the Official View is undermined by this sentence. Nothing is defined. One big word – 'compassion' – is thought to be explained by other big words: 'care', 'empathy', 'respect', 'dignity' and 'intelligent kindness' – which are also not defined. The statement also seems to make some sort of factual claim – that 'compassion is central to how people perceive their care', without any valid evidence to support it.

In fact, it's not even clear what 'compassion is central to how people perceive their care' means. Does it mean that a certain number of people regard compassion as an essential component of care – that care cannot take place without compassion? Does it mean that people who were asked what care means to them mostly cited 'compassion'? Or does it mean that most care includes compassion as a matter of fact? It's just not clear.

Cummings' 6Cs were taken from work in the 1980s and 90s by Simone Roach, who was interested in what nurses actually do while they are caring for others. Roach's list of Cs was essentially descriptive, identifying behaviours she saw in practice and that she felt could helpfully indicate what nursing is (22). Her list contains 7Cs, some of which were directly copied by Cummings (strangely without reference or acknowledgement of the source) (23). For reasons she does not explain, Cummings chose to omit some of Roach's Cs. The most telling – and troubling – omission from the Roach list is:

> Creativity
>
> Creativity is having a vision of how nursing care can be, and making it better. Creativity in nursing requires thinking reflectively, critically and imaginatively to create healing environments and enhance caregiving practices. It requires the nurse to develop the qualities of envisioning, risk-taking, openness and resourcefulness. Creativity results in integrating new insights into existing nursing knowledge and awareness. It creates the potential for the nurse to individualize care and embrace change. (24)

Unlike Roach's, Cummings' list of Cs is prescriptive – this is what we think nurses should do. Were she to have included 'creativity' it would have been a better list, emphasising autonomy and imagination and signalling the need for a less mechanistic educational environment. But unfortunately our current times increasingly require conformity over adventure, and most of our present leaders, in all social spheres, lack the will and imagination to stand up for human inventiveness.

This aside, Cummings surely means 'compassion' to be a central value for carers – as well as a required attitude and behaviour. However, unless you specify what 'compassion' means and doesn't mean, you're actually not offering any practical, meaningful guidance. 'Compassion' isn't an obvious emotion – what's it like to 'feel compassion', and how can we tell if we are feeling it? It's not obvious what compassion is in any particular circumstance. Is it compassionate to give money to a beggar, or is it guilt? Is it compassionate to give to charity, or is this really just a way to feel good about ourselves? Is it compassionate to 'go the extra yard' at work, or is this merely the best way to get a promotion or salary increase?

'Compassion' can mean one behaviour to one person and a different behaviour to another person – even a completely contradictory behaviour – which means that generalised advice to 'be compassionate' is useless. One person might think 'being compassionate' means going along with everything a patient says whereas another may think it compassionate to challenge the patient, even to be cruel to her, to be kind in the long run. Affirmation and cruelty – both could be compassionate, in exactly the same circumstances.

It should be quite obvious that a few words, inexplicably beginning with the same letter, really aren't any use to anyone: 'courage' for example could mean the courage to blow the whistle on bad practice or it could mean the courage to go into work every day, despite the bad practice, to put food on the table for your children.

All the 6Cs are open to debate. Values aren't like flat-pack furniture instructions, or a car repair manual guide – they're entirely different in kind. In case any doubt remains, consider this actual case. There are any number of real situations that reveal the emptiness of advice to 'follow a C', but the case of Betty and Derek is especially compelling. If you wish, you can browse to the issue on this book's Values Exchange, offer your own response, and see what everybody else thinks: http://thoughtful.vxcommunity.com/Issue/betty-and-derek/23053

 STOP & THINK TWO: BETTY AND DEREK

Betty and Derek are both in their eighties, and have been living in a residential home for the past nine years in separate rooms. They have always had a very close marriage and do everything together.

Betty suffers with severe bilateral macular degeneration and as a result can see very little and is registered blind. She also has very poor hearing and has used a wheelchair since her arthritis became severe a few years ago.

Derek has been very ill with pneumonia. His health has deteriorated significantly over the last few days but he refuses to be admitted to hospital, stating that he wants to remain where he is and, if it comes to it, wishes to '...die with Betty present, holding her hand.'

At 3am Derek deteriorates rapidly. His breathing becomes laboured and shallow as his respiratory rate drops. The carers wake Betty from her sleep. Unfortunately, while taking Betty to Derek's room, there is a medical emergency and the nurse who is pushing Betty has to stop, to run to help with it.

Sadly, in the time it takes for the nurse to return, the carers discover that Derek has passed away. The carers consider their options, which include telling Betty that Derek is still alive, allowing her to sit and hold his hand for a while, and then telling her he's passed away a little later, taking into account her blindness and hearing problems.

Would that be the compassionate thing to do? Can it be compassionate to deceive, or does 'being compassionate' require that the truth be told?

It is proposed that the carers lie compassionately to Betty, telling her Derek is dying rather than dead.

Add your response on the Values Exchange: http://thoughtful.vxcommunity.com/Issue/betty-and-derek/23054

(With thanks to Vanessa Peutherer, VX Learning Facilitator, for this example.)

What is the compassionate choice in this case? To lie or tell the truth? Both actions are arguably compassionate – but not everyone will agree on what's truly compassionate. What's the caring or committed thing to do here? Benign deception – maybe risking your job – or scrupulous honesty – risking further devastating the elderly Betty?

Are Values Really the Basic Problem?

Because values are so widely referenced and discussed it seems to many commentators that eliminating 'bad values' and promoting good ones is an effective way to improve social systems. The idea seems simple enough: if we weed out people who have 'the wrong values' and empower those who have 'the right values' then surely things must get better.

This is exactly what Robert Francis QC assumed in his review of the Mid Staffordshire Hospital scandal (25, 26, 27).

The Mid Staffs Scandal

Between January 2005 and March 2009 hundreds of hospital patients died as a result of substandard care and staff failings at two hospitals in

Mid-Staffordshire, England. Some patients received the wrong medication or no medication; receptionists rather than doctors decided which patients to treat; nurses switched off equipment because they didn't know how to use it; and there was pressure to meet arbitrary targets set by NHS managers, including a 4-hour waiting time limit to treat people in Accident and Emergency (28).

According to the *Daily Telegraph*, the scandal is thought to have occurred because managers attempted to cut costs and meet targets for caring for patients within certain time limits, in order to achieve a coveted 'foundation status' for the Trust.

These targets apparently ruled supreme, overriding any other considerations, including personal judgement. NHS managers staffed the hospital so thinly that there were never enough consultants to supervise junior doctors adequately, so the juniors took their instructions from senior nurses and matrons, who religiously enforced the targets. Orders were cascaded down the management hierarchy – and nurses and doctors who failed to meet them were threatened with the sack. Junior nurses and doctors were repeatedly forced to abandon seriously-ill patients to treat minor cases who were in danger of breaching the 4-hour Accident & Emergency waiting time limit. And patients were often moved out of Casualty covered in their own excrement because the target – to admit or discharge patients within four hours – was under threat.

In the public inquiry, Francis identified an 'unhealthy and dangerous culture'. The Francis Report highlighted a failure in many cases to 'put the patient first', and pinpointed several common characteristics of NHS hospital trusts which contributed to this failure including: a lack of candour; low staff morale; disengagement by medical leaders; and cultures of inward-looking secrecy and defensiveness (29).

Francis made 290 recommendations, intended to be systemic and aimed at preventing a recurrence of the scandal. However, his main reform idea was that the NHS should operate according to a common set of values and standards, with tools to measure whether or not they are attained. He also recommended a process called 'values-based recruitment' (VBR) – a mechanism to appoint people with 'the right values' by using psychological tests and asking them what they would do – or what they actually did – in situations which seem to require a 'caring approach'.

Values-based Recruitment

Following Francis, 'values-based recruitment' is now being implemented by universities and the NHS, though not without some well-justified scepticism (30). Either by asking potential recruits to say how they would act in challenging situations, or by asking them to describe real life situations in which they have made value judgements, it's thought to be possible to screen out bad applicants (31).

The programme is led by Health Education England (HEE) (32) which references the National Skills Academy (NSA) as an example of good practice. The NSA recommends that 'the easiest way to find out about someone's underlying values is to ask them about how they behave in their everyday lives' since previous behaviour is the best predictor of future behaviour, and suggests asking candidates to give evidence for their behaviours. Some general interview questions are offered as possibilities, for example:

> Could you give me an example of a time when you have had to work with people who have required different levels of support or assistance.
>
> - How did their needs differ?
> - How did you accommodate these differences?
> - What was the outcome?
> - What is important to you when caring for another person?
> - Why do you think it was important to them?
> - How does it make you feel when you hear about people being mistreated and why do you think this happens sometimes? (33)

Superficially, values-based recruitment makes some sense, but give it any sort of thoughtful reflection and its weaknesses are overwhelming. The **NSA's** questions – and any other question-based way of scoring people's personalities – are hopelessly flawed. The method is unable to detect if candidates are being honest in their answers, discover if candidates' responses change over time, match candidates' responses to actual behaviours once the person is recruited, or assess the impact of respondents' values on the patient care they actually deliver. These are hardly insignificant drawbacks.

Not only this, but experimental psychology tells us that in many circumstances (though not all) many of us will cheat, steal and lie while at the same time seeing ourselves as honest, upstanding citizens (34). Whatever values we say we have, we know scientifically that if we can get away with it – and if we will still feel our integrity is intact – then we will merrily act on opposite values to the ones we claim.

Worse still, officially:

> Values-Based Recruitment is an approach which attracts and selects students, trainees or employees on the basis that their individual values and behaviours align with the values of the NHS Constitution. (35)

But as we've seen already, the values cited in the NHS Constitution are vague, ill-defined, contestable and impossible to apply without controversy so – quite frankly – trying to 'align individual values' with 'the values of the NHS Constitution' is like trying to catch a shadow in a dream. It's just not possible – and the fact that so many expensively educated people think it is, is disturbing.

The Values Epidemic

It's not just in the ultra-labelled world of the NHS that values are misunderstood. It's rare to find any organisation that fails to declare it's values these days. Yet, without exception, these declarations are generalisations and bluffs – just as they are in the NHS. Organisations consist of complicated people and complicated relationships, rules, systems and strategies. They are just not the sort of entities that can act on simplistic values, even if they wanted to. Thinking of organisations as a simple unit, with plain, straightforward values is an extreme delusion, as any example will show.

The Coca Cola Company – a soft drinks manufacturer and distributor – says it 'lives its values' in everything it does:

> Our values serve as a compass for our actions and describe how we behave in the world.

Coca Cola's values apparently include:

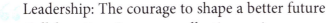

> Leadership: The courage to shape a better future
> Collaboration: Leverage collective genius
> Integrity: Be real
> Accountability: If it is to be, it's up to me
> Passion: Committed in heart and mind
> Diversity: As inclusive as our brands
> Quality: What we do, we do well. (36)

Coca Cola claims it values 'integrity' yet in practice there are many who question its ethics, pointing to worker exploitation, water shortages caused by its overseas factories, extensive lobbying of politicians to allow genetically-modified ingredients, misleading advertising and obesity exacerbated by the high sugar content of its products (37, 38).

For some reason Coca Cola believes it is able to muster 'collective genius' (what's that?). And that it, and presumably every one of its individual employees, exhibits commitment in 'heart and mind' (it's not clear to what).

Yet its primary value is very obviously missing. Coca Cola exists to make a profit (it has a net worth of $180 billion) yet its list of supposed values would sit equally well with a not-for-profit charity (39).

Every organisation from the biggest health authority to the smallest sports club uses 'values statements' in an equally empty fashion. MacDonald's restaurant, for example, has this list:

> McDonald's brand mission is to be our customers' favorite place and way to eat:
> We place the customer experience at the core of all we do.
> We are committed to our people.
> We believe in the McDonald's System.
> We operate our business ethically.
> We give back to our communities.
> We grow our business profitably.
> We strive continually to improve. (40)

Of course McDonald's wants to be its customers' favourite place and way to eat, and wants to increase its profits and the rest. But this is only a part of what makes McDonald's tick. To find a more genuine picture watch the following short video clip (41): www.youtube.com/watch?v=B3swf0Sj5bc.

The item contends that far from operating ethically, McDonald's appeals to simplistic patriotism; glorifies war; is the second worst paying company in the US next to Walmart with an average full-time wage of only US$18,000 (in 2016); intimidates staff who try to organise union activity; makes employees pay for and professionally clean their own uniforms; offers bizarre advice on budgeting, including a suggestion to get a second job; costs the US public over $1 billion in public assistance (food stamps for instance) because it does not pay adequate wages for families; sticks salt all over children's Happy Meals in order to make them thirsty and so buy more of its sugary soft drinks; and is the second largest purchaser of beef in the country, supporting cruel factory farming without conscience.

No-one would seriously expect McDonald's to say it values low wages, intimidation and animal abuse – even though it quite plainly does, because these are its preferences and it's the preferences we act on that show what our values really are.

'Positive values' are paraded in every sector. Even the British Army has a list:

 Everyone in the Army should aspire to the six core values and standards of the British Army:
Loyalty
Integrity
Courage
Discipline
Respect for others
Selfless commitment (42)

There's little doubt that to be a soldier requires all of these qualities one way or another, but as they stand they are just words, with no substance, stated apart from any practical context. In fact, they're so imprecise that any organisation could happily adopt them – the British Army's list would be equally helpful to Al Qaeda or Isis or The Salvation Army or the Boy Scouts. For 'values statements' to have any real meaning at all, each 'value' requires definition and elucidation by examples.

What sort of loyalty does the Army require: blind or thoughtful? I once had a heated conversation with an Army Chaplin who considered himself an 'ethics expert'. We were talking about the ethics of warfare. His view, it emerged, was that if you are in the Army then you should not think about the causes of, or the justice of, any conflict you happen to be in. Basically, as a soldier, yours 'is not to reason why, yours is but to do or die'. By joining the Army, you apparently agree to any rules it had when you joined – even if you were unaware of them – and also agree to any future rules and orders, whatever they are, even to consent to actions that are likely to kill innocent civilians. The Chaplin and I finished up discussing Gallipoli, a pointless conflict over possession of a rock in World War I in which over 46,000 soldiers lost their lives (43). At one point in the fighting, a British commander ordered Australian and New Zealand soldiers to climb out of a trench into fierce gunfire and almost certain death. I asked whether the soldiers' duty was really to do something so utterly insane, and he replied that they were ethically committed to do so, out of duty and loyalty. I replied that in my view this had nothing to do with ethics and everything to do with extreme control, arrogance, callous stupidity and the intolerable abuse of power. I remember saying that ethics begins when we're able to think for ourselves, not when we are so scared or indoctrinated that we will face death rather than challenge blatant idiocy. Our conversation came to a rather abrupt end when I told the Chaplin that a much more ethical approach to the situation would have been for the trench soldiers to shoot the British commander between the eyes.

If you exhibit blind loyalty, then where is your integrity? If you have sacrificed all your choices then how can you exhibit any integrity, maturity or autonomy? And what sort of courage ought you to exhibit: the courage to do whatever you are told by your commanders or the courage to say no to orders that you find immoral? Certainly, it would take courage to endanger yourself according to a ridiculous order from a superior, and it would take courage to refuse. And because these would be different forms of courage, and require totally opposite actions, it's worthless to say that a single world – 'courage' – is a 'core value and standard'. It's just not credible to do this when the same word can be applied to competing actions.

So yes, we can all agree in principle that it's important to 'respect others', and I'm sure members of the British Army regularly do so. But at the same time we need to understand how 'respect for others' squares with decades of bombing campaigns in the Middle East and elsewhere, specifically intended to kill or maim tens of thousands of other human beings. Where does 'respect for others' begin and where does it end? Are there more powerful values – like for example winning wars or selling weapons – that can trump 'respect for others', and if there are how do these operate? Even more important, why can these values trump other values? What is the ethical justification for this?

To answer these questions, we need to get rid of lists of values. They can be one useful starting point for deeper discussion, but if they go unchallenged they become barriers to thought.

Unfortunately, the idea that it is enough to write out lists of words in order to assure yourself that you are 'ethical' and have 'the right values', is taught to us as very young people. Schools, which you would hope might know better, have their own lists of 'values'. There's hardly a laudable concept that some school or other does not lay claim to, in fact they seem to be in informal competition to see which of them can select the most audacious: 'excellence for all', 'inspiration', 'going beyond the possible', 'being all you can be', 'changing the world as we know it' (truly) – so why is it that in practice schools rarely if ever achieve these aims? Why is a quite different set of values routinely acted on? And why – despite the evidence to the contrary – do most parents and teachers imagine that only fluffy, positive values are the real drivers of schools' behaviours?

Here's a typical school example:

> Our Vision and Values
>
> We believe that all children have the right to the very best education. Our aim is to provide this by ensuring that our core values of respect, care, honesty, responsibility, friendship and determination underpin everything we do. (44)

This particular school, like hundreds of others in the UK, says it upholds 'British Values' as well as its own:

> ... the British Values of DEMOCRACY, THE RULE OF LAW, INDIVIDUAL LIBERTY, MUTUAL RESPECT and TOLERANCE OF THOSE OF DIFFERENT FAITHS AND BELIEFS are embedded within our school. (The school's capitals.)

But none of these shiny values is consistently acted upon. If they are applied simultaneously they often conflict in practice, and contradictory values are routinely exhibited. For example, I might value individual liberty and at the same time claim the right to be intolerant of people (of different faiths and beliefs) who do not believe in individual liberty. Or I might – as a pupil – be determined to come out on top, in competition with my friends, wanting to beat them. And how is it respectful to children to force them to go along with a system designed to classify a significant proportion of them as 'failures' or as 'needy' or 'inadequate'. Doesn't this really exemplify gross disrespect?

And in what ways are schools actually democratic?

Why don't we see this on school websites?

> Our Vision and Values
>
> We believe all children need to conform to our particular education system. Our aim is to ensure this through a process of indoctrination that lasts for well over a decade for each child. Regardless of their interests, abilities or desire to learn the limited range of subjects we offer, we grade and measure children so they can eventually leave school with certificates and awards (or, in the case of the many children our values damage, leave with no certificates and a record of underachievement). We expect all children to accept our values and priorities even if they have different values and priorities of their own. Our values underpin everything we do.

This would be at least as accurate as the Official View, and it rests on values just as much, but would obviously never be owned by a single school. Conformity, acceptance, rule-following, mindless tradition, school priorities over child priorities – these are more central to schools than 'liberty', 'tolerance' and 'respect': yet they seem to be a dirty secret, forever absent from 'values statements' and 'school missions'.

It's downright confusing and frustrating. On the one hand schools say they are creating rounded, curious, fearless, free-thinking citizens, on the other their only measure of success is how well they teach students to pass exams and get good grades.

This **STOP & THINK** is a simple survey, not a Think Screen. It was set up, in the public domain, by a school teacher and responded to by school students. The original data are retained. You can see these if you respond yourself.

> **STOP & THINK THREE: SCHOOL PRIDE, GOOD OR BAD?**
>
> Is School Pride a virtue or a vice?
>
> Virtually every school has an inspiring motto (often in Latin), meant to set it apart from others. Most schools have distinctive uniforms, signifying belonging to that one school rather than all schools.
>
> Many schools actively try to foster School Pride through chapel and assembly, and by celebrating student achievement. This is meant to create a sense of belonging and identification with the school's values.
>
> Even within schools, many schools have 'houses' and similar systems, encouraging pride in a specific part of the school.
>
> Is this the way things should be? Is it right and noble to have pride in your school above all other schools?
>
> Or can you have too much pride? Is promoting School Pride in some ways counter-productive? Does it perhaps create a sense of tribe against tribe? And is this a good message for later life?
>
> Add your response to the Values Exchange: http://thoughtful.vxcommunity.com/Issue/school-pride-good-or-bad/13335

A Very Strange Delusion

There is something very strange going on here. The leaders of pretty much every organisation, large and small, not only think it essential to announce a handful of their 'Sunday best' values to the world, they also believe that doing so makes a positive difference.

Almost everyone seems certain that the **Official View** is true (there are a few exceptions (45)). Almost everyone's sure values are fundamental to the way we choose to act – and everyone's convinced lists of undefined words can consistently inform individual and institutional activity. But just because everyone thinks something is the case doesn't make it true.

Values-based recruitment is extensively used, in various guises, as an employee selection tool. Indeed, the majority of higher education institutions are using some form of values-based recruitment for NHS-funded training courses. The idea has quickly gathered so much traction that it's now commonplace for applicants to prepare lists of their use of the 6Cs before their interviews, carefully rehearsing examples of their courage, commitment and compassion. However, despite widespread deployment, there's no standard model for the use of values-based recruitment, and as yet no evaluation of its efficacy (46).

> VBR assumes that recruiting for values and behaviours, and then maintaining and encouraging these, will improve the quality of healthcare provision. Whilst intuitively appealing, there is no evidence to support this assumption. The evidence that exists is unsystematic and largely anecdotal. There have been no evaluations of the impact of VBR on aspects of care such as 'compassion' or variables such as staff retention rates or indicators of organisational health (such as staff sickness and absence rates). (47)

Take a minute to think about this. Values-based recruitment is widely practiced within a system that prides itself on evidence-based practice and rigorous research, but no-one in any of the universities or health authorities that use it has a clue if it has any validity or brings any benefits. For all we know values-based recruitment might be harmful. It certainly is to those whose employment prospects have been damaged by it (48).

Worse still – much worse in my opinion – is that you don't even need evidence to know that values-based recruitment can't work. Health Education England says values-based recruitment is an approach which aims to attract and select health care students, trainees or employees 'on the basis that their individual values and behaviours align with the values of the NHS Constitution' (49). But as we know, the values of the NHS constitution are misty and mysterious – they are certainly not solid or specific enough to be meaningfully aligned with anything.

Nor do you need evidence to know that the Official View of values is superficial. Values are not what the establishment thinks they are. This is a matter of fact.

Here's the Official View again, with brief comments in italics:

1. Values can be clearly differentiated from each other – *no they can't: is it courageous or compassionate or caring or committed or competent or an example of good communication, to lie to Betty about Derek's lonely death? Can't it be all of these things, or a combination of them, or none of them, or some other sort of choices? In reality what we value is mixed up and complicated. It's artificial to see values as separate, stand-alone preferences.*

2. Values can be held and exhibited both by individuals and organisations – *values can be held by individuals, there's no doubt about that, though values are not held in separate chunks. However, organisations cannot exhibit values – other than in the rules and policies they lay down to be followed – because values are preferences and preferences require a subject to hold them. Organisations are nothing more than groups of people working together for some goals, consistent or otherwise. It's the individual people who make the decisions, and it's their preferences and choices that create the organisation.*
3. Values can be clearly identified as consistent drivers of individual and organisational behaviours – *this is not true because values are indistinct and can be interpreted very differently by different people. And in any case, values are not the fundamental drivers of behaviour – there are far deeper forces at work.*
4. Values expressed as single words are understood in the same way by everyone who reads or hears them – *this is obviously untrue. Of course we can mostly agree what words like 'honesty' and 'respect' and 'dignity' mean in general, but both in theory and in practice people understand them in different ways. Does 'honesty' mean always telling the absolute truth about everything or does it mean something more complex, and more interesting? Is an 'honest person' only a person who favours total disclosure regardless of the negative impacts this might have, or can we say that an 'honest person' is generally trustworthy, reliable and can be depended upon to make thoughtful, caring judgements about what information to give and what to withhold? And after all, in health care, health workers are required not to tell the truth all the time (which in a sense is dishonest), in the interest of maintaining confidentiality.*
5. Lists of different values – often known as 'values statements' – can consistently guide the actions of individuals and organisations – *this is false because of the imprecision of the words and because once a more specific meaning is given to them, the more detailed values inevitably begin to clash in practice.*
6. People can and should be recruited according to their values – *people can be recruited according to what they say they value and according to what they do. Some of these statements and behaviours will reflect some preferences, but these preferences can change at any time, and in work situations there are frequently more powerful influences in play than values.*

7. If an organisation professes the right values it will make the right decisions – *simplistic lists of values are mantras, they don't guide organisations' decisions in any meaningful way. Organisational decision making is multi-layered, political, thorny, often controversial and – as everyone knows – different members of organisations can disagree profoundly about what to do – and yet they are all supposedly guided by the same values.*
8. Lists of values help us tell the difference between right and wrong – *absolutely not. Ethical decision making is rich and complex and influenced in all manner of ways, most of which we are unaware of. It is we individuals that decide what is right and wrong every time we make a choice, regardless of any list of values.*

This is an immensely daunting set of misconceptions, which surely requires some explanation. How can so many intelligent people so badly misunderstand the nature of values?

Values as Labels

When people are blind to truth that should be staring them in the face, we have to ask: why can't they see it? What's hiding the deeper reality of values from all the people that advocate them?

I can't prove this – this isn't science – but I think it's predominantly a problem of labelling. Values words and statements are frequently used as labels. People and organisations like to wear them on their sleeves – or perhaps tattoo them on their arms. In this form, most values claims are little more than insubstantial bravado: 'we value integrity', 'we put people first', 'we respect everyone', 'Kevin loves Sharon'. Because so many people use values in this way, it seems everyone is unwittingly deluding each other, and few feel the need to peel off the labels to see what's really going on.

Labels are designed as a form of display and as a way of offering summary information – this is an Audi or a Ben Sherman or a best-seller. They're meant to be taken at face value: if it's an Audi you can trust it's mechanics, there's no need to look under the bonnet. That's the first problem. The second – and even more deluding problem – is that labels give the impression that everything is separate: this is an Audi, not a BMW; we value 'integrity', 'loyalty' and 'dignity' but not all the other values we might have listed. In these two ways, labels shrink our perceptions, diminish our curiosity and foster a culture of passive acceptance.

Ultimately, Little Bits of Reform are Not Going to Work

There really is a fundamental problem here: if you try to change the world under a delusion, it isn't going to work. Changing superficial labels is nothing more than changing the colours of the deckchairs on the Titanic. Reform after reform makes one recommendation after another and yet everything stays pretty much the same, or even gets worse. As Richard Vize has commented:

> [After Francis] … with a government anxious to claim it was putting patient safety first, and something approaching a moral panic in the health service about adequate staffing of wards and a fear among managers of them becoming the next Mid-Staffs, there was a rush to employ nurses beyond the capacity to supply them. This triggered an uncontrolled expansion in spending on agency staff, which has played a substantial role in driving the NHS into a financial crisis. (50)

Change one thing, apparently separately, and you'll have an impact on something else. You might not intend or foresee it, but it will happen. It's simply a law of economics – and until we start looking at the world in a richer way, it will never end.

And this is precisely the case with values-based recruitment too – and to be honest this was more than a little foreseeable. A focus on the individual in an incredibly complex environment is simply not going to deliver. As Susan McPherson and Syd Hiskey have noted:

> With the current emphasis on recruiting and 'training' staff to be more compassionate, little focus has been placed on barriers (both structural and interpersonal) that undermine staff compassion. A study of frontline staff working on dementia wards found that staff have intuitive ways of responding compassionately. But the realities of the workplace, such as styles of management and unsympathetic structures, often prevent them doing so. A focus on compassion training and Values-Based Recruitment therefore seems misguided without a parallel commitment to removing barriers to compassion.

The focus on measuring the compassion of possible NHS employees, via a Values-Based Recruitment process, bears little resemblance to the recommendations Francis made. His report emphasised the 'systemic failings' in Mid-Staffordshire. In this sense, the NHS system is woven into the very political and social fabric of the United Kingdom. (51)

Francis' idea to align practice with NHS values does sound plausible, until you start to ask meaningful questions. How am I, as a student doctor or nurse, to demonstrate the 'right values' in reality rather than in an interview that I have prepared for? How do I know what the 'right values' are in any real social situation? How do I even know what my own values are? How do I know what other people's values are? How do I know what my clients' values are?

If I seem to have 'the wrong values' how can I improve? Assuming it's possible to understand my clients' values, how do I handle situations where what I value is not the same as what my client values?

How do I deal with values conflict? How do I react in circumstances where my clients' values are opposed to mine? How do I cope if I am in an organisation whose stated values are not the same as mine? What do I do if my organisation says it espouses a list of values, but in reality acts on different values?

What Values Really Are

There's no doubt that values are a meaningful concept, but they don't exist in the concrete fashion that almost everyone thinks they do.

The word 'values' is really nothing more than an indicator that some being – a human, another animal, even a plant – likes something.

'Values' can indicate a preference for some grand ideal – millions of people prefer Western democracy over dictatorships, so we say that they 'value democracy' (or that democracy is one of their values). But 'values' do not have to be the big, impressive-sounding words we see in so many mission-statements – rather the word 'values' purely refers to anything that's preferred over something else. If I prefer eating tofu to eating meat (which I do) then I value eating tofu and I disvalue eating meat: 'eating tofu' is a value of mine and 'eating meat' is not. The same applies to black coffee over latte, strawberries over cream and using a touch screen computer rather than a standard desktop.

Most plants prefer sunlight over shade, so it makes sense to say of my sunflowers and tomatoes that they value sunlight and that therefore sunlight is one of their values. This may sound a bit strange, since we do not usually think of plants having values – or that sunlight can be a value – but it's a perfectly logical conclusion.

All living beings have an extraordinary array of values – not just the 'big ones' like freedom, dignity, rights and equality. And because life is in constant flux, values are not fixed – they can change just as any desire can change over time and through experience. Many years ago – as a very young man – I did eat meat and had never heard of tofu – but now I know better. I now have a whole set of other values that feed into and support my choice not to eat other creatures that have emotions and purposes. I doubt it, but it's possible that one day my values will change, through some shift in knowledge or a change in my circumstances. Think about your own values – big and small. Look back and see how they have changed as you have changed, and notice too that they have not changed spontaneously, but as the result of the complex backcloth to your life, your growing and the world around you changing and influencing you in fresh ways.

Note too that we rarely hold our values consistently – though of course we think we do, until we examine ourselves closely. My partner – Vanessa – is resolute in the values she believes in, but one day was surprised to find that she was completely contradicting what she thought was her fundamental preference: the right to know – to be informed in order to make your own choices. As a nurse these values are quite basic to her philosophy of care, but as a mother it turned out that in some circumstances they can swiftly be ditched. We were on an Air Malaysia flight travelling from Kuala Lumpur to London, when one of the engines began to leak fuel. The captain explained that we would have to return and land in Kuala Lumpur, but first we needed to circle for an hour or so in order to ditch fuel so that we could land safely. Vanessa's son, Zak (then 11), was asleep all this time and – in order to protect him – she decided both not to wake him but also not to tell him anything about what was going on, should he wake. She simply could not bear to frighten him or to see him fearful so she withheld the information, in complete contrast with what she supposed her fundamental values were.

This **STOP & THINK** is a simple poll – and also a perfect way to interrogate our values.

STOP & THINK FOUR: SECONDS FROM DISASTER

The crude combination of a kitchen timer, paper and cardboard found in a lavatory on an Air France flight could have been a bomb, but the crew didn't tell passengers of that possibility. Instead, people were told the plane had a technical problem and would be landing in Kenya instead of Paris.

Sunday's decision, which was short of the full truth, raises an ethical question about when passengers should be fully informed of problems in the air. But many experts say the crew of Air France Flight 463 did the right thing, avoiding panic and quickly landing the plane. Once on the ground, security officials determined that the device was a hoax, and passengers were told the full story.

'We pay our captains to make good decisions and you've got to back them up,' said Robert Mann, a former airline executive who now is president of R.W. Mann & Company, Inc., an airline consulting firm in Port Washington, New York. 'In this case I think the crew made a really rational decision.'

He said the crew had no evidence that the device was an actual bomb, so telling passengers there was a technical problem was true 'in the sense that they didn't know what they had.'

The Boeing 777, originally headed to Paris from the island of Mauritius, was diverted to Kenya's coastal city of Mombasa. Hundreds of passengers left the plane on emergency slides. Afterward, several praised the flight crew for keeping everyone calm.

Most airlines don't have hard-and-fast policies on what to tell passengers, leaving that up to the crew, according to Alan Price, a former chief pilot for Delta Air Lines and founder of consulting firm Falcon Leadership. Here's the article in full: www.miamiherald.com/news/nation-world/world/article50830135.html.

One argument is to not disclose the true nature of an emergency until the plane has landed safely as this will be the best option for keeping the passengers calm, especially given once airborne there is nothing passengers can do to ensure their own safety.

The other argument is that because of this lack of personal control passengers deserve to know the truth, as they ought to know the likelihood of a dire outcome so they can personally prepare, and in some instances where connectivity allows, be able to contact loved ones on the ground.

Most of us have been airline passengers. If an emergency is taking place in the cockpit, would you want to know the truth or something else?

What do you think?

It is proposed that passengers should be fully informed of problems in the air.

Add your response on the Values Exchange: http://thoughtful.vxcommunity.com/Issue/think-stop-four-seconds-from-disaster/23055

(Issue originally created by Amanda Lees.)

Not only does values inconsistency happen to everyone, it's bound to happen to everyone because reality is messy. Several scholars have come up with hierarchies of values (52) where values are ranked – often in quite complicated systems – but these simply have no bearing on reality, they are just some academic's fantasy. When, for example, we talk about rights we tend to talk about the rights that work for us, not those that work for others. If we're rich then we are likely to claim a right to our wealth, but if we suddenly become poor we are sooner or later more likely to advocate for more egalitarian rights – it's just a fact of life.

Seen in their proper light – values are not concrete attitudes that can be taught or adopted easily. Values are part of a fluid tapestry of preferences, influenced and movable in many ways of and beyond our choosing – by genetics, our families, our experiences, our psychological type, our physical and mental capabilities, our reflective learning, our changing circumstances and so on – our values are at the mercy of our restless lives.

Let's end this chapter with a collective experiment that proves the values delusion.

Simply ask yourself: What are my values?

You can write out a list if you like, but that isn't the way to discover your values. In fact, your list is likely to be a delusion. You will most likely write out what you think your values ought to be, not what they actually are.

Instead, think about an apparently simple situation, and what you would do. As you think, take note of how you feel and what thoughts directly occur to you.

This is the situation. It's happened to most of us:

STOP & THINK FIVE: THE BANKNOTE IN THE BUSH

You are walking out of your workplace and all of a sudden you see a bank note.
  Is it your lucky day? What do you do?
  You have several options, of course: take the money for yourself, just walk past leaving the money, take the money to a police station, take the money to the workplace reception, take the money and donate it to charity, take the money and give it to your hard-up friend, or maybe do something else …
  Which of these options exhibits 'the right values' – they surely can't all do so, so which are the right ones and which are wrong?

> You can either think about it privately, discuss it with colleagues or friends, or you can respond online.
>
> Add your response on the Values Exchange: http://thoughtful.vxcommunity.com/Issue/think-stop-five-the-bank-note-in-the-bush/23056

Initially you'll probably be unsure what to do. You will most likely experience some internal conflict, but you will rationalise this and come to some position you can justify. You will also discover, by looking at everyone else's answers, that there's external conflict too. Like pretty much any social decision, what to do about finding a bank note in the bush is controversial. People make all sorts of different choices and offer all sorts of different justifications. Essentially, people apply a wide range of values in conflicting and inconsistent ways to address even the most apparently simple situation.

Fortunately, we are on the way to understanding why: superficial labelling, artificial separateness and a lack of will to think more deeply.

Beneath the labels – beneath the apparent separateness of things – there's a rich, complex and partly unknowable sea of feelings, logic, beliefs, truth, falsehood and inconsistency. It's quite possible – simultaneously – to be respectful and intolerant, loyal and dishonest, inclusive and discriminatory, compassionate and angry, profitable and socially aware, to seek excellence while punishing failure – and any other combination of values and priorities. We all know this since we all act on conflicting values every day.

We think values are solid and separate because this allows us to talk about them. For example, we often assume that 'caring' is a single, separate value that means the same thing to everyone in all contexts. However, this just isn't true. In order to handle the complexity of values we fashion them into something artificial – we create a form of reality, but it is at best a poor shadow of deeper truth.

We do the same thing with all our concepts – social and scientific. We do it with education, rights, history, animals, risk, health, school, ethics – you'll find many examples in Chapter 4. And we do it with ourselves too, both in the way we think of ourselves and in the way we think of other people. The **Bank Note in the Bush** case is a very basic illustration of the depth which underlies our simplifications.

Most people, before they start to think about the bank note conundrum, imagine they will be able to decide easily since they assume they are good people with good values. Most people also assume that most other people will choose the same answer as them, and offer similar justifications. Yet in reality most people – not all, admittedly – find it hard to decide what to do and pretty much everyone is surprised to see the diversity of the results. We don't all think the same – far from it.

There is an easy view of reality that says 'honest people who have the right values will do X for reasons Y' and then there is a much more complex and puzzling view of reality that says: 'people who think they are honest will do many different things for many different reasons in an apparently simple situation involving a bank note in the bush – and we are not really sure why one person does one thing and another does a different thing.'

If we are to make better decisions and create policies and reforms that actually work, then we need to understand that nothing is really the way we have made it look. We create a superficial view of social life – a sort of wilful mirage, a self-induced hallucination of orderliness and sameness. We'd rather think things are easy to understand than accept the truth that nothing's easy to understand. And we'd rather think we are all more or less the same –and think that we all experience roughly the same reality – than work with the truth that everyone of us experiences a different reality.

Even though we use the same labels, nobody sees the same world as everyone else.

{ SUMMARY OF CHAPTER 1 }

1. Officially, values are considered to be solid attitudes that are consistently acted upon, and which can be prescribed and taught. But the Official View of values is almost entirely mistaken.
2. Thoughtful examination of the NHS Constitution shows this beyond any doubt.
3. The 6Cs are a further example of the deluded over-simplification of reality. For example, health workers are urged to be 'compassionate' but 'compassion' is a complex and intricate concept, open to wide interpretation. And in practice, actions one person would define as compassionate are often defined as 'lacking compassion' by other persons – and there is no way to prove one person is right and the other wrong.

4. Values-based recruitment (VBR) is officially regarded as a way to prevent callous practice, but reality is far too multifaceted to make this anything more than fantasy. For example, VBR is unable to detect if candidates are being honest in their answers, discover if candidates' responses change over time, match candidates' responses to actual behaviours once the person is recruited, or assess the impact of respondents' values on the patient care they actually deliver.
5. There is a values epidemic that affects almost all contemporary institutions, from McDonald's to the Army. These institutions mirror the values delusion in the NHS, their leaders not only think it essential to announce a handful of their 'Sunday best' values to the world, they also believe that doing so makes a positive difference. But the values epidemic is nothing more than a symptom of shallow thinking.
6. Values words and statements are frequently used as labels. In this form, most values claims are little more than insubstantial bravado: 'we value integrity', 'we put people first', 'we respect everyone', and so on. Because so many people use values in this way, it seems everyone is unwittingly deluding each other, and few feel the need to peel off the labels to see what's really going on.
7. Values are a meaningful concept, but they don't exist in the concrete fashion that almost everyone thinks they do. The word 'values' is really nothing more than an indicator that some being – a human, another animal, even a plant – likes something. 'Values' do not have to be the big, impressive-sounding words we see in so many mission-statements – rather the word 'values' purely refers to anything that's preferred over something else.
8. 'Values' is not a fundamental concept, despite its current popularity. Values or preferences are caused by many complex factors in the environment, in our psychologies, in our belief systems, in our emotions, in our histories, and so on.
9. Values are not fixed. People's values are a rich mix and which is most dominant in any decision can fluctuate for all manner of reasons. Values are much less stable and predictable than is generally believed. For example, in similar circumstances a person can be honest one day and dishonest the next.

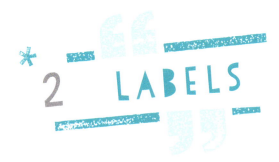

2 LABELS

A fundamental limit on the way we understand the world and each other is our need to label everything. Labelling is like a spotlight. It brightly illuminates a small part of the stage, but leaves everything else in shadow.

Nothing is Obvious

We like to think everything has a simple explanation – we just need to find it. Then we can label it and put it in its rightful slot on the reality shelf.

Why did we lose the soccer game? Why did that car accident happen? Why did my relationship fail? Why did I burn the toast? Why did those patients die unnecessarily? Why did my boss act aggressively towards me? Why did the rocket ship explode? Why is our climate changing?

When we ask such questions, we're driven to identify THE cause. There it is. There's your trouble. Our forward line's not tall enough. The driver lost attention. My wife is a psychopath. The toaster's too cheap. It was a failure of care. My boss is a psychopath. It was a fuel leak. It's CO_2.

Why, just for example, did that road accident occur? One car ran into another at the traffic lights. What was to blame? Who was at fault? What caused the incident? What can we do to prevent it happening in future?

The traffic lights changed. Jim moved forward; Jenny was behind him and moved forward too. All of a sudden Jim stopped abruptly. Jenny's car ran into the back of Jim's car. What was the cause?

The insurance company said it was Jenny's fault. She should have been more attentive. The police agreed – especially since Jenny had two toddlers in the back. THE cause was that Jenny was too distracted and when Jim stopped suddenly she didn't react quickly enough. But was that really THE cause?

Jenny had been out the night before. She was a little hungover. Her children were playing a 'screaming game' in the back. One of Jim's brake lights was not working. Jim stopped abruptly because a dog (not Iggy!) ran across the road in front of him. The dog's owners dropped the lead because they were arguing about money. Their bank had just refused them a re-mortgage. Their bank manager fancies the male dog owner. The bank manager is gay but won't admit it to anyone, not even himself. Because he's frustrated he tends to take it out on his objects of desire, which made it easier for him to refuse the bank loan. The traffic lights had just been serviced and were operating slightly differently from their normal phasing. Jenny's brakes are worn because she can't afford to change the pads. Jenny was made redundant six months ago. Jenny's previous employer gambled in stocks and shares. The share market collapsed …

Which of these – and which of the infinite number of other connected factors – is THE cause?

When you think about it, to ask for THE cause makes no sense. Of course it's possible to create flow charts that culminate in what you suppose is THE cause. But how do you decide what THE cause really is, when everything is so interrelated? Choosing THE cause of anything complex is an arbitrary judgement. We could play with labels. Talk about direct and indirect causation. Degree of causal responsibility, and so on. But that's just us oversimplifying, in order to make a sense of things in a way we can handle. Reality is far deeper than our convenient summaries.

It's probably easiest to blame Jenny, but was she truly THE cause? Isn't it just as likely that it was the Bank Manager's fault? Imagine the Bank Manager was not gay, was not feeling hard done by and decided to allow the dog-owning couple's mortgage. Had that been the case the dog would not have run across the road and there would not have been an accident. Don't you think?

Of course it sounds ludicrous to say that the cause of a road accident was a bank official's covert homosexuality. Yet that is surely no more ludicrous than to say that the basic cause of the accident was Jenny's lack of care.

The real truth is we don't know what caused the accident, but we can't accept this. We need to pin down some plausible explanation, so we can breathe a sigh of relief. That's what it was. We'll make sure it doesn't happen again. It's labelled now. Phew.

The problem is, as we identify THE cause we do a lot of other things too. We pick one reason out of a multitude of other possible reasons. We attach a label – which says THE cause – to that reason. We don't attach the label to the other possible reasons. So we separate out one reason from all the rest, because that is what we are psychologically determined to do. This, we decide, is a special reason. It's not like all the rest. It's THE reason.

STOP & THINK SIX: THE OPEN WINDOW

Rachel (a woman in her twenties) was badly disfigured in an accident. She had been depressed.
  Rachel had previously told hospital staff she was considering suicide.
  Today she fell to her death from an open hospital window.
  There was no suicide note.
  In your opinion, what was the basic cause of her death?

Add your response on the Values Exchange: http://thoughtful.vxcommunity.com/Issue/think-stop-six-the-open-window/23057

Seeking 'the basic cause' in a sea of complexity is the perfect example of the ceaselessly controversial act of labelling the world.

We seem unable to accept that most things are too complicated to explain. Who knows what caused Rachel to fall from the window, it could have been so many factors or combinations of factors. To nail it down to one or two is plainly artificial.

Seeking to identify 'the core problem' is a reasonable approach to relatively simple challenges, for instance if you jump into your car one morning and it won't start. Since a car is a closed system made up of interacting parts there's a finite list of why this should be – no petrol, flat battery, faulty starter motor, broken ignition switch, engine flooded with petrol, and so on. Through a process of elimination, it's quite possible to uncover the 'root cause': is there petrol in the tank? Does the engine turn over? What happens if you replace the ignition switch? Is it the carburettor?

But most of the world is not made up of closed systems, and in any case even closed systems interact with other closed systems effectively creating open systems (like the cars involved in Jim and Jenny's road accident). Families, work places, people's lives, hospitals, schools, universities, jungles, parties, disputes between people, human relationships – all of these are unpredictable, open systems where even if you fix what you think is the 'key fault' they will evolve as they will. Open systems cannot be fixed in mechanical ways.

Trouble is, the Francis Report (and the hundreds of similar efforts over the years) thinks of the NHS like a car with a faulty carburettor when it is really an astonishingly complicated human village, and must be understood as such if we are to make any real sense of it.

Francis' recommendations are typical of the 'Official View' of the world. He sees everything as distinct, objective, definable, separate and concrete – even very vague and elusive ideas and concepts. As a lawyer he's spent a lifetime working with definitions and rules, so it's hardly surprising he thinks like this, but it doesn't make him right.

Understandably, Francis assumes that there is an external reality that's the same for everyone. If that external reality is a problem then it can be fixed by deliberately changing the parts of it that are problematic, he says.

We're all very used to this view of the world – it's the one politicians, policymakers and managers pay homage to all the time.

> We can fix this. We know what the problem is. We've identified the cause. We've put our finger on the basic faults. We have recommendations. We can reform the system and the problem will disappear. We are the experts at fixing these things.

Wrenches and screwdrivers at the ready, politicians and policy reformers advise:

> There's your trouble. It's the carburettor. We think you need a different one. That one's no good anymore.

> There's your trouble. It's the way the system's organised. We need to create internal markets. We need to create commercial incentives. We need to treat health care like a business. And here are 357 specific ways we recommend to do that.

It is easy to have sympathy for this approach. Sometimes it works. Just as treating a patient like a machine to be fixed by therapy X or Y sometimes works. But it doesn't always work. It often backfires, even if it says it works on the label.

Flags

Pasting simple labels over depths we are not equipped to understand is bound to lead to trouble.

The most obvious example of the point and peril of labelling is our unstoppable urge to colonise other lands and other peoples (we're still doing it – as of 2012, 16 territories with a combined population of over 2 million were deemed to be under colonial rule (53)).

Whenever we colonise, we quite literally stick labels on the world, as we use our flags to lay claim to pieces of it.

The flag is a universally recognised symbol of possession. The act of pinning a coloured canvas to a piece of earth, or maybe to a significant building standing on a piece of earth, has a staggeringly powerful effect on us, quite out of proportion to what any calm appraisal should tell us. Pin a flag on a territory and all of a sudden the territory's nature seems to change.

American astronauts even put a starched stars and stripes on the moon.

James Cook, a much-lauded scientist, cartographer and explorer, was an inveterate labeller of land – indeed the countries he explored and claimed for the British Crown are themselves now littered with the label 'Cook'.

The following brief account of Cook's first landing in New Zealand appears in a chapter entitled 'These People Are Much Given to War' in *Cook: A Biography* by Richard Hough (54). Hough writes:

> It took almost three days and nights to close this coast, so unfavourable were the winds. But at last, on the afternoon on 9 October, Cook manoeuvred the *Endeavour* into a wide bay and was able to report:
>
> "We saw in the bay several canoes, people upon the shore and some houses in the country. The land on the sea coast is high with white steep cliffs, and inland are very high mountains. The face of the country is of a hilly surface and appears to be clotted with wood and verdure."
>
> It all looked so promising, almost as if they were off the chalky Sussex coast …

Hough continues:

> Cook ordered the pinnace (small boat) … to be launched … soon after they landed on the river bank, they saw a small party of Maoris [sic] on the other side, so they re-embarked and crossed over to confront them … Cook, Banks, Solander and Midshipman John Bootie followed them as far as a collection of huts, all empty. "We then went up and examined one of their houses," Bootie recalled, "which we found to be low and very close and warm, thatched after the same manner as our houses in England."

I've read this particular passage many times and I am never less astounded by the psychology of it. The seamen found land that looks like home, they could clearly see that it is farmed and inhabited, and they discovered cosy dwellings with familiarly built roofs. And yet at the same time, their first reaction is not only to stick a flag in the ground to claim it for England, but to confront the natives, seeing them as alien and dangerous, despite the obvious humanness of their residences. (In fact, as it turned out, the white people were far more dangerous to the 'natives', their muskets shooting and killing six Maori in the space of two days, before they decided to beat a judicious retreat.)

The comedian Eddie Izzard puts his finger on it. How do you build up an empire, he asks?

Answer:

> We stole countries with the cunning use of flags.
>
> I claim India for Britain!
>
> You can't claim us, we live here. 500 million of us.
>
> (In a haughty, plummy, British tone) 'Do you have a flag? … No flag no country … that's the rules that I've just made up …' (55)

An oversimplification, as many hundreds of scholars will tell you, but hardly a complete oversimplification. One of the most effective techniques for taking over other people's countries is to relabel them. Knock down their statutes and stick up some of your own. Put your flags on their castles. Simple.

Louis Althusser – a French Marxist philosopher – had a slightly obscure theory called 'hailing'. The idea is that a flag, or some other powerful symbol, somehow captures the individual viewing it, in a way well beyond reason. As he or she is 'hailed' she confuses her own identity with the flag:

> Ideology "acts" ... in such a way that it recruits subjects ... (56)

We all know the impact of flags during times of national crisis or success, for example during international soccer competitions, when flags appear everywhere like flotsam. It's a kind of collective hysteria, where people's powers of judgement disappear under a welter of gaudy bunting.

Sticking a flag in the ground is one of the simplest acts human beings can do. But as every indigenous, colonised people knows all too well, the act of labelling their land has the devastating effect of hiding most of, if not all, their history, culture, language and traditions. What the label stands for privileges just one of many ways of social life, concealing so many fascinating differences that would enrich everyone's lives.

STOP & THINK SEVEN: ARE YOU PROUD OF YOUR NATIONAL FLAG?

Flags create a sense of identity and unity. Flags also create a sense that all nations are different from each other.
   Use this very short survey to connect with others to debate the effect of flags.

Add your response on the Values Exchange: http://thoughtful.vxcommunity.com/Issue/think-stop-seven-are-you-proud-of-your-national-flag/23058

The Packet Trap

In one way, our ability to label is a blessing, particularly since it allows us to communicate threats and opportunities to each other. But labelling comes with a big price.

Ernst Cassirer, a twentieth-century German philosopher interested in the philosophy of culture, contended that while other animals perceive their world through their instincts and direct sensory perception, we humans create our own universe of what he called symbolic meanings – symbols of every kind that act as a double-edged sword; helping us interpret our sensory perceptions in ways that are meaningful and helpful to us, but at the same time putting increasingly thick barriers between us and 'reality in the raw':

> Physical reality seems to recede in proportion as man's symbolic activity advances. Instead of dealing with the things themselves man is in a sense constantly conversing with himself. He has so enveloped himself in linguistic forms, in artistic images, in mythical symbols or religious rites that he cannot see or know anything except by the interposition of [an] artificial medium. (57)

It's possible that Iggy, the labrador we met in the meadow, is freer than we are. Iggy may see more variety and possibility in the meadow than we do because his mind is more open – less cluttered with meanings. Iggy may have fewer preconceptions than we do. He has no words and uses no symbols. Iggy is more likely to be surprised by the meadow than we are, just as we were when we were children.

When we were youngsters meadows were astonishing places. Full of stories and legends shared amongst friends; saturated with strange sounds and smells and colours. Meadows were places for games and fantasy – for imagination and for collecting flowers and leaves and rocks and excitement. Each time we entered the meadow we felt anything could happen – it was up to us to make it so.

But as we begin to make sense of things with our adult labels – honour, success, sin, disgrace, right, wrong – we start to freeze our view of the meadow. Because we're social beings who use a shared language, our constant use of the same set of meanings becomes a habit. And the more we're habituated the less inclined we are to ask questions.

We're all familiar with this effect. Describe a child as a 'gifted athlete' or as 'rebellious' or as 'suffering from ADHD' or as 'obese' or as 'backward' and that's typically how he or she will be seen. Not only that but each label will bring other labels with it, reinforcing the main one. The 'obese' child, for example, is likely to be seen as 'lazy' or 'greedy' or 'exercise-shy' or 'lacking will-power', but these are just a few of many possible labels. The child is much less likely to be seen as a victim of aggressive marketing by fast food companies or the meat industry, simply because this label is currently less used.

It's impossible to overestimate the power of labels. Call a person a 'rebel' or a 'fanatic' or a 'genius' or 'unpredictable' and it's as if they have a tattoo on their forehead that instructs us to see them and their actions in certain ways and not others.

There's a moment in the classic film *One Flew Over the Cuckoo's Nest* where the inmates commandeer a fishing boat. They are all in the boat, preparing it to leave. At first, they appear as unusual (you might even say 'as insane') as they do in the asylum. Then something magical happens. McMurphy (Jack Nicholson) is challenged by an official who wants them all to get off the boat. He introduces them:

> We're from the state mental institution …,

a revelation which seems about to curtail their expedition,

> … this is Dr Cheswick, Dr Taber … Dr Scanlon – the famous Dr Scanlon …

and so on.

With just the change of one word – Doctor for Mister – the inmates transform, and all thanks to the power of labels (58).

In one infamous study, researchers entered mental hospitals as patients, but behaved as normally as possible. However, because they were officially labelled as 'schizophrenic', even the most innocuous behaviours were interpreted as caused by their imagined mental illness (59). Once the label 'mental patient' or 'schizophrenic' is attached to a person, any behaviour – even the most ordinary – is attributed to the 'illness' (60).

It takes a real effort of will to see past labels. Once a person's labelled 'a fanatic' it becomes very much harder to think of him as anything else. There doesn't seem to be much room left for other labels: 'loving father', 'devoted son', 'man of faith', 'great cook', 'kind to his pets' and so on, yet the 'fanatic' may well be all these things – a complex human being with a complex life, just like everyone else.

We've categorised reality into our packets throughout history, convinced that the labelling we use in our particular era is true for all time – while forgetting the vast historical evidence that whatever labels we have faith in now will sooner or later be rejected, as we reconsider what we know.

This is strikingly clear in health care, where our beliefs about nutrition, ethical practice, infection control, health promotion, mental illness and much else, are constantly revised and redefined. In the 1950s, smoking was barely seen as a health issue, in the 1960s meat was regarded as essential to good health and in the 1970s homosexuality was considered a mental illness (61, 62, 63).

Eventually, most of our labels end up contradicting each other. Even something as seemingly simple as a window or a vase of flowers get totally contrasting labels slapped on them.

According to Florence Nightingale, adequate ventilation – which for her meant opening windows as much as possible – is the very first canon of nursing (64). Yet to some current hospital managers, an open window is an unacceptable health and safety risk. In 2012, for example, all the windows in a new wing of the Victoria Hospital in Kirkcaldy, Fife were locked in case staff and patients fell out of them (65).

Nightingale labelled flowers in a very positive way, describing the 'rapture' of patients with fever on seeing a vase of brightly coloured flowers. Possibly anticipating the modern day ban on flowers in hospital wards (see Chapter 4), she sternly admonished the 'folly and ignorance' which cause experienced nurses to 'leave the patient stewing in a corrupting atmosphere' with windows tightly closed while 'denying him, on the plea of unhealthiness, a glass of cut flowers or a growing plant' (66).

> This is a plant pot, it says so, on the label. It's a pot for growing plants in.

But the plant pot can have so many other labels. It can be a discussion piece, a work of art, an ornament, a bird's nest, a home for ants or kittens, a weapon, a present, any colour you like, a toilet, a sanctuary for a tortoise or a mouse, a holder of fire, something to paint, something to be smashed up and used as hard core for concrete, a musical instrument, a subject for an essay or a poem, an illustration in a book on delusions, fancy dress, a cooking vessel, a prize in a raffle …

A plant pot is just for plants only if we want it to be. A difficult patient is a difficult patient only if we label her that way. A risk is a risk only if we say it is. A celebrity is a celebrity only if we believe the labels our shallow (spot the label) culture sticks on people. A scandal is a scandal only if we choose to be scandalised.

STOP & THINK EIGHT: POSITIVE OR NEGATIVE?

Choose one object, event or behaviour and give it two labels: one positive and one negative. Which label is true?

 Add your response on the Values Exchange: http://thoughtful.vxcommunity.com/Issue/think-stop-eight-positive-or-negative/23059

Separateness

Labels fool us into thinking that the world is made up of parts which have only a passing relationship to each other.

It's as if everything – ourselves included – consists of little packets of reality, fenced off from other packets, and labelled compulsively. We even see ourselves as built out of separate packets – 'I'm really nothing more than a collection of molecules, cells and tissues'; 'back then I was a different person'; 'I'm a fireman/policewoman/undertaker/academic/comedian/journalist/INSERT YOUR OWN JOB TITLE HERE' (rather than anything else); 'I don't let my feelings cloud my judgement'; 'It's all in the past, I've made a totally fresh start'; 'I never bring my work home with me', and so on. It doesn't matter what aspect of life we consider, with only the slightest effort we're able to parcel it up and file it in the appropriate cabinet, losing sight of the innumerable connections that make us the bafflingly complex beings we are, becoming numb to the unfathomable relationships buzzing everywhere in nature.

Our overwhelming urge, when we view infinite richness – an ocean, a rainforest, a petri dish full of microbes, the sky at night, a child asleep, a lover's eyes – is to reduce it to something we can understand, and cope with. This is certainly not unique to health care – it's a universal human tendency. We have an inexorable aversion to mysteriousness. We're constantly seeking certainties – it hardly matters whether they are true or not.

As the interesting musician Moby has written:

 The world is too big and too intricate to conform to our ideas of what it should be like. In my experience I've found that most fundamentalists aren't so much attached to their professed ideologies as

> they are to the way in which these ideologies try to make sense of a confusing world. But the world is confusing, and just because we invent myths and theories to explain away the chaos we're still going to live in a world that's older and more complicated than we'll ever understand. So many religious and political and scientific and social systems fail in that they try to impose a rigid structure onto what is an inherently ambiguous world … if we base our belief systems on the humble assumption that the complexities of the world are ontologically beyond our understanding, then maybe our belief systems will make more sense and end up causing less suffering. (67)

It's no use reassuring ourselves with make believe. If we're ever to be more sensitive to each other and the swirling disorder, we need to recognise mystery for what it is, wherever it is. And we need to accept it. We need to roll with it, not try to mould it into detached silhouettes.

We Can See Things as Separate if We Want To, But Do We Want To?

It's possible to read items of news as if they are separate from any other item of news. It's possible to believe events occur randomly without any deeper patterns. It's possible to define illnesses in separation from other parts of the body or mind or environment. It's possible to see each other as mysterious strangers.

Seen one way we certainly are separate. Seen one way events do just happen. If I drop a book on my toe, then its only my toe that hurts. If I feel a stab of sadness then it is only I who feels that pain. If my luggage is stolen, then it's my loss to bear alone. But this is just one way to look at the world. If it's a delusion – as I'm sure it is – then if we continue to try to fix our problems only with this assumption, we are bound to fail.

Ultimately it doesn't really make sense to look at any aspect of the world – natural or human – as if it is disconnected. All you have to do is consider any individual life, even briefly – the connections are inescapable.

We all had parents. Most of us in the developed world were fortunate enough to be looked after by them, at least for a while. We inherited our parents' genes; we learnt from other people, from books written by other people, from events organised by other people. Someone else made our clothes; someone else grew our food; someone else mined the coal that warmed us; someone else drilled for the oil that powered the trucks that brought us the coal, and clothes, and food. Someone else fought wars that enabled the political system we grew up in; someone else picked me up when I fell off the push bike someone else built for me and someone else bought for me, and sat me gently in his van to take me home, made by bricks and mortar and expertise that I had no idea about whatsoever, but which if not there would have been part of a different personal life.

There was, in the late 1970s, a documentary series that – like most else in this book – has, for reasons I do not understand, stuck in my mind. The series was written by James Burke. It was called *Connections*, and thanks to digital technology it's available today for anyone with a computer and internet access. Burke's simple and compelling idea was that 'progress' is not a step-by-step process where one improvement precedes another separately, in succession, rather it's a delusion (my word) to consider the development of any particular piece of the world in isolation.

According to Burke, our modern world could not be what it is without a vast web of seemingly separate events actually being connected. Burke repeatedly shows that unless X happened in 1661 (or some such date) then Y could not have happened in 1967.

Burke's view is that unless technological inventions, which were always his examples, are seen as connected to other inventions then we do not see them correctly. To demonstrate the point, Burke begins each episode with an event or innovation from the past and then traces a path from that event through a sequence of apparently unrelated connections to an indispensable aspect of the modern world. For example, Burke's *The Long Chain* episode traces the invention of plastics from development of the fluyt, a type of Dutch cargo ship. Other episodes suggest that modern telecommunications exist because Normans had stirrups for horse riding (*Distant Voices*) and that the Little Ice Age (c. 1250–1300 AD) was responsible for the invention of the chimney, knitting, buttons, wall tapestries, glass windows and the practice of privacy for sleeping and sex. Burke's point is that any change inevitably causes more change: if someone invents a windscreen for a car then someone else is bound to invent windscreen wipers and washers, and if a new technology is required for this then a snowball effect ensues. To use Burke's own examples: if you start with the plough you get craftsmen, a form of civilisation, irrigation, pottery, mathematics, calendars (to account for the seasons and predict floods) 'and a modern world where change happens so rapidly you can't keep up' (68).

Everything seems separate only if we see it that way. To see this all you have to do is look at a picture of a rainforest. You could see the entire picture as one complex reality – seeing abstract colours and patterns. But you will most likely see trees, plants – maybe birds – as separate items because this is your expectation. You will see discrete objects that you put together to make up the picture.

But we always have options: separateness or connectedness, which is it to be?

You can see veins on a leaf. Or the leaf. Or a tree. Or a wood. Or a landscape. Or a whole globe. Each are views of reality. You can choose which view to adopt: packets or threads.

If everything is endlessly connected to everything else, then the world is much more mystifying than we can comprehend. We should stop pretending that it isn't.

STOP & THINK NINE: CONNECTED OR SEPARATE?

Think about your life. All you have done. All that has happened. All the stuff you know. All the people you have met. As much as you can.

The poet Maya Angelou once mused:

'I've learned that people will forget what you said, people will forget what you did, but people will never forget how you made them feel.'

Thinking about your life, do you feel connected or separate?

Add your response on the Values Exchange: http://thoughtful.vxcommunity.com/Issue/think-stop-nine-connected-or-separate/23060

We Label Our Problems

We label our problems too. In fact, without labels we cannot have any problems.

Here's the pattern.

Step One: somebody must decide that something is a problem, or not. Losing a ticket to an opera is a problem if you're anticipating a musical treat, but it isn't a problem if you're looking for an excuse not to go. The unexpected death of a protected tree in your garden might be a disaster if you are a plant connoisseur but a blessing if you need extra space to park your car. Being deaf is a problem if you want to hear, but not if you're a proud member of the Deaf community. Becoming terminally ill is a problem if you want to live but, if you've had enough of life, it's a gift.

Step Two: because of our obsession with labelling, the problem must be seen in a certain way – it's not just any problem, it's this sort of problem rather than that one. For example, consider Paul, who's not doing well at school. We might say that Paul is a problem because he's not working hard enough to achieve pass grades, or that the problem is Brian who's an incompetent teacher, or that the problem is the personal relationship between Paul and Brian, or that the problem is the whole school because it's not delivering a sufficiently stimulating education, or that the problem is the entire education system whose scope is too limited, or even that the problem is made up of most or all of these factors. But however we see it, it's we who define the scope and scale of the problem. Problems do not frame themselves.

Step Three: any attempt to solve the problem will focus on the problem as we've defined it, rather than any alternative way we might define it. For example, rather than see Paul's attitude as troublesome, we might instead decide that there is something wrong with the way adults think of children. We tend to believe children need to be taught, need to learn to think like us, need to adopt our priorities and need to be equipped to live lives similar to the lives we are living ourselves. But maybe they don't. Maybe the problem is our view of childhood. It's up to us to say.

Think about the problems you have right now.

It doesn't matter what the problem is, nor does it matter how big or small it is – it has to take the three step shape outlined above: just try to find a problem that doesn't.

Perhaps take a very small problem: you have a jar of olives but the lid is stuck. Try as you might you can't get it off. Then ask yourself why it's a problem. What made it a problem in the first place?

The only possible answer is that somebody (in this case you) identified the stuck lid as a problem. The problem didn't create itself. The jar of olives is what it is. Its lid becomes a problem only if you want to open the jar.

If, for example, you wanted to exhibit the olive jar in a museum, or place it in a time capsule, or use it as a decorative ornament, or paint a picture of it, or photograph it, or give it as a present, or travel with it secure in the knowledge that the lid won't leak, the fact that the lid won't come off is irrelevant or even a good thing.

But you want to eat the olives, the jammed lid is a problem – according to you. In some circumstances the stuck lid doesn't matter. In other circumstances – always defined by you – the lid is a problem. And always, how big a problem it is, is also up to you.

Five essential questions should be constantly in mind, not least if you are a health professional: What is the problem? Who says it's a problem? To whom is it a problem? Why is it a problem? How much of a problem is it?

I'm in Health – How Does Thinking About Labels, Separateness and Packets Help Me?

It may be difficult to see how the knowledge that we stick our labels everywhere is of practical help to health professionals and health professional students. After all, most of us rarely think about labels. If anything, we unconsciously take refuge in them and the certainty they offer. But as the examples in this book accumulate, it should become clearer and clearer that seeing the world as separate parcels limits our imagination, awareness and creativity.

The child diagnosed with ADHD, for instance, may be helped to calm down by Ritalin (the preferred medical therapy for his disease label) but he will always carry the diagnosis of mental illness with him; his boredom and need for a different form of stimulation other than school will be ignored; his qualities – his brightness, his energy, his desire to challenge authority – will be seen as deficits; and his questions and enthusiasm will be regarded as cheeky, mischievous and disruptive. A little may be gained but much more will be lost. See the boy with just one set of labels and the rest of him vanishes from view.

We all need to stand back from the daily grind to see behind the standard rules and instructions of working life, to become more aware of the complexity and connectedness of everything, and to develop strategies to think independently of the labels that signpost almost every aspect of our lives.

If everything around us is really technicolour and we're only looking at it in black and white, then we're not seeing enough. As a consequence, the ways we deliver health and social care will be less rich and less imaginative than they might be. If we care with blinkers on we're bound to miss creative, life-enhancing opportunities – and enhancing lives is the very heart and soul of health and social care.

As we will see in the next chapter, our labelling is only one part of a veil between ourselves and reality. We assume we all see the same world – and we assume as well that our view of life and other people is accurate. But this too is a myth – a comforting blanket, not the truth.

Once you are aware that there is so much more to daily reality than meets the eye, you can never turn back. But you will be a far more inventive health worker as a result.

SUMMARY OF CHAPTER 2

1. Labelling is necessary for us to define the world around us and to communicate with others.
2. However, our need to label also limits the way we understand the world and each other. Labelling is like a spotlight. It brightly illuminates a small part of the stage, but leaves everything else in shadow.
3. It's impossible to overestimate the power of labels. Call a person a 'rebel' or a 'fanatic' or a 'genius' or 'unpredictable' or as 'having ADHD' and we're immediately inclined to see them and their actions in certain ways and not others.
4. It takes a real effort of will to see past labels. This is strikingly clear in health care, where our beliefs about nutrition, ethical practice, infection control, health promotion, mental illness and much else, are constantly revised and redefined. In the 1950s smoking was barely seen as a health issue, in the 1960s meat was regarded as essential to good health, and in the 1970s homosexuality was considered a mental illness.
5. Labels fool us into thinking that the world is made up of separate parts which have only a passing relationship to each other. It's as if everything – ourselves included – consists of little packets of reality, fenced off from other packets, but this is a false belief. It is the packet trap.

6. Ultimately, it doesn't make sense to look at any aspect of the world – natural or human – as if it is disconnected. All you have to do is consider any individual life even briefly – the connections are inescapable. It is particularly important, if you are a health worker, to see your patients in this light.
7. It may be hard to see how the knowledge that we stick our labels everywhere is of practical help to health professionals and health professional students. But, as the examples in this book accumulate, it will become clearer and clearer that seeing the world as separate parcels limits our imagination, awareness and creativity. We all need to stand back from the daily grind to see behind the standard rules and instructions of working life, to become more aware of the complexity and connectedness of everything, and to develop strategies to think independently of the labels that signpost almost every aspect of our lives.

3 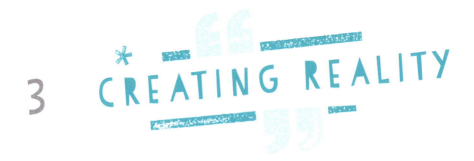 CREATING REALITY

There is absolutely no doubt that in all sorts of ways, the way things appear to we human beings is not the way things really are. It's simply not possible for us to access pure, unadulterated reality. Everything we receive from the world outside us is filtered by our senses, our beliefs, our education, our era, our sciences, our technologies. No-one sees exactly the same world, because no-one is the same as anyone else. Iggy's world is not – and never can be – my world. Neither can my world ever be yours.

The idea that there's no single true reality is commonplace to professional philosophers and many other academics, yet it can seem rather peculiar when it's first encountered. Thankfully, many scholars have worked hard to explain it, including Bertrand Russell – a twentieth-century English philosopher – and still one of the clearest popularisers of philosophical puzzles.

In *The Problems of Philosophy*, a book aimed at the general public, Russell devotes a chapter to appearance and reality, systematically challenging the 'common-sense' view that we all see the same world (69).

He describes a simple scene:

> I am now sitting in a chair, at a table of a certain shape, on which I see sheets of paper with writing or print.

Apparently stating the obvious, Russell comments:

> I believe that, if any other normal person comes into my room he will see the same chairs and tables and books and papers as I see, and that the table which I see is the same as the table which I feel

pressing against my arm. All this seems to be so evident as to be hardly worth stating ... Yet all of this may be reasonably doubted, and all of it requires much careful discussion.

Russell points out that any sensible person is likely to agree that the table looks brown, oblong and shiny; to the touch it feels smooth, cool and hard; tap it and it gives out a wooden sound, and so on.

Yet one by one Russell shows that each of these apparent facts is easily called into question.

We naturally assume that the table is just a single colour, yet open-minded observation quickly refutes this. Russell describes a walk around his table, reporting that he can see different colours dependent on his point of view. Some parts of the table, for example, reflect more light than others, causing different shades of brown to appear.

Anyone can confirm this at any time. Carefully scrutinise any object you think is a single colour and you'll see. At first you'll very likely insist it really is just the one colour – a brown table, a red chair, a black computer – but look a little more closely. Walk around it like Russell – or simply move your head slightly – and you will see that some parts not only look brighter than others but are different shades. Shine a torch on a part of the object and that area may even appear white. What's more, if several people are looking at the object from different angles (as they must be since we all occupy a unique position in space and time) then no two of them will see exactly the same object.

We quickly reach a fundamentally important and far-reaching conclusion: the colour of the table is not caused only by the table itself – as a separate thing – but by a relationship between the observer, the table and what Russell calls 'the external conditions' (for example, the way the light falls on the table). The observer has visual capabilities (which are dependent on how good the observer's eyesight is). She has a physical point of view (where she is standing, how near she is to the table, whether she's moving or not). The table is made up of atoms and molecules that can change their arrangement. And the external conditions can vary considerably: is the room that houses the table in light or darkness? Is the sun shining or is it cloudy? Are lamps reflected in the surface of the table? and so on.

Russell challenges the idea that one real colour of the table even exists. Instead, he says, when we talk about the colour of something we tend to refer to some usual perspective of it (the table in the afternoon light, for example). But there's no reason to assume that this usual perspective should be considered real and other perspectives should be considered less real. Why do we not assume that the colour of the table under other conditions is the true colour (the table at 1a.m. in the morning, for example). Why should the most usual brown be considered the true brown of the table, to the exclusion of the other browns, or even other colours, that sometimes appear?

And it's the same with texture, Russell explains:

> … to the naked eye, the table appears to be smooth and hard. Aided by microscope, the grain of the wood enlarges to appear as a mountainous range of different roughnesses and textures.

Why should one impression of the table's texture be thought of as more real than another?

Russell argues that we are not struck by these discontinuities in our daily life because we learn 'to construct the "real" shape from the apparent shape …'. We come up with an ideal version of the table in our minds, and this ideal version overrides what we actually see.

As Russell explains, while for practical purposes these differences are unimportant:

> … to the painter they are all-important: the painter has to unlearn the habit of thinking that things seem to have the colour which common-sense says they "really" have …

Instead, the painter must learn to see past inattentive common sense to notice the subtleties of light and perspective that are presented to him. To paint with accuracy, the painter has to escape the delusion that the way things appear is truly the way they are.

Once this realisation sinks in it can be quite a shock. Just as it came as a shock to us as babies when we discovered that hiding our eyes didn't make us invisible and that objects that leave our field of vision don't really go out of existence.

Once you accept that the way things seem to you is just one of endless ways to see reality, it's like a dam bursting. While Russell's point is pure philosophy, the implications for health care (and everything else we think we understand) are immense.

Most of us view health care as a hierarchical, rule-governed, partly science-based human system intended to help people affected by disease and illness. Typically, within this system, clinicians are the experts, health is the opposite of disease, budgets are balanced to prioritise 'health needs', ethics committees dictate what is right and wrong, and policies are defined at the top of a managerial pyramid.

But if Russell is right (which of course he is) this is just one way the health system – and its goals – is offered to us. The system is not necessarily like this. If we apply Russell's method to it, we can see it in deeper ways. And we can act within it as we think best, if we want to.

We can accept the health system like a health official, or we can perform within it like creative artists.

Our Reality is Created by Relationships

This is such an important finding. It is hard to overstate its significance. No-one sees exactly the same world. We may receive the same information, but the impression we have access to is a result of the relationship between the data we receive and our own interpretation of it – and in turn this interpretation is affected by every part of us: physical, psychological (transference and projection, for example (60)), emotional, historical, political – every part of us.

We can see the world only with our own eyes and understand it only with our own knowledge and experience – no-one else's.

Is this a frustration? None of us can get past our own perceptions of reality, and none of us can ever be sure that the way we see things is the way other people see things. It could seem a lonely prison.

But surely it's more liberating than entrapping. Once you appreciate the true situation, it frees you up. You are, for example, far better placed to try to understand what other people are experiencing, thinking and saying. You know for sure that the way you see it will be different – possibly completely different – from the way they do. You also know that the way they see things – just like the way you see things – is caused by an exclusive combination of the external world and them; which gives you constant opportunity to try to work out what perceptions and reasons other people have.

In health care, to give a simple and accessible example, if you don't think hard enough you may conclude that a person who is petrified to receive an injection is a 'coward' or a 'wimp', afraid of a 'scratch' that you deliver daily to many patients. But if you ask instead, 'How can it be that this person is so frightened?', 'What is it in her perception of the needle that makes the reality of the needle for her so intimidating?' then while you may never know for sure you will at least be open to seeing the world closer to the way she does, rather than projecting your view of the needle – and of her – on to her. She may be hypersensitive to physical pain (70). She may have a phobia of needles (71). She may have had a previous bad experience with an injection or another medical procedure – she may even have forgotten this but it may still be affecting her. She may have a child who was damaged by a needle – or maybe had an adverse reaction to a vaccination. She may have recently seen a documentary or a horror film or talked to other patients about needles. There may be many reasons for her fear that you do not know, but which you may take the trouble to find out, now you understand that reality is a relationship, and therefore different for everyone.

Russell's approach may seem abstract, but it can be applied to any aspect of our lives with powerful effect. Used intelligently and with empathy this philosophical insight has immense implications for daily health care. To grasp more of this power of awareness, simply substitute 'hospital' or 'the patient' for Russell's 'table'.

What is the Real Hospital?

As Russell has explained, each of us will see, touch and smell a slightly different hospital – dependent on our physical perspectives. Each of us will see a different hospital in other ways too, dependent on our knowledge, our personal history, our culture, our age, our physical and mental condition, our personality, and so on. And this raises fundamental philosophical and practical questions: what is the real hospital? Is it the same hospital to different people?

All the different aspects of being in hospital combine, in different ways for each person, to create a rich, complex and unique array of experiences, making 'standardisation' seem less and less realistic (72).

Is it the same hospital to the senior surgeon as it is to the 15-year-old child with cancer? Or to his parents and siblings? Is it the same hospital to Sarah, the confident, career focused young nurse as it is to Catherine the 73-year-old grandmother, diagnosed with Alzheimer's 30 minutes ago?

If you look upon the architect's blueprint for the hospital, there is – quite obviously it seems – just one hospital made of specific materials with certain dimensions. It has wiring and piping and fire escapes and elevators – and they are all in the same place for everyone. In this sense there is only one building – and in a fire, everyone will, if they possibly can, all head for the safest exits.

But this is only one way to look at a hospital, or any other object or process or person in the world.

Think of a patient. If the patient is your mother, you will see her not as your brother does but as you do – just like your unique view of Russell's table you will have a unique view of your mother – she will be reflected in all the ways in which she is connected to every aspect of your being.

The patient does not exist to you separate from your understanding of her. Reality is not separate from us.

STOP & THINK TEN: THE REAL THING?

Think of any object, event or person you like. Consider its appearance. Consider its purpose. Consider its qualities.

Which of these would exist if you were not observing it?

Add your response on the Values Exchange: http://thoughtful.vxcommunity.com/Issue/think-stop-ten-the-real-thing/23061

Is it the same hospital to Sarah and Catherine?

Sarah's Hospital

Sarah is a 37-year-old nurse. She has worked in the hospital for her whole career. She's just been appointed as a nurse manager – a very significant promotion for her. She's excited and happy with her life. To her the hospital is home – she knows almost every nook and cranny, and every corner she turns a different – almost always happy – memory springs into her consciousness.

When Sarah approaches the entrance of the hospital she is optimistic, confident. It's as if the hospital has its arms outstretched to greet her. She can't wait to get inside and do her job.

Even when she touches the walls or work tops or hangs up her gear in her locker everything is familiar to her – it's almost as if the hospital is part of Sarah. And in a way it truly is because so many of her thoughts and memories are to do with the hospital, and if we are not constituted by our thoughts and memories, what makes us who we are?

Catherine's Hospital

Catherine has never been to this hospital before. She has been on the site however – at an old hospital demolished 23 years ago. She gave birth to her first child in the old building – she can recall that perfectly. But this new place is harsh to her, stony and repelling. The walls are ugly and cold and they make her feel like an alien.

At this moment she's walking unsteadily out of the hospital, along a corridor so long and shiny it's making her pulse race with nervousness at the glare of it. Her daughter – Annie, her first child – is holding her hand and her arm. That feels good to Catherine, in the starkest contrast to the hospital itself.

Catherine has just been told she's losing her mind. That her memory is draining from her body – that her very self is vanishing. She can't take all that in, but somehow she knows it's true. And if she has to forget then she definitely wants to forget that she's losing herself. It is unbearably painful to her.

For some reason Catherine has suddenly become hyper-sensitive to sound. Every noise – every metallic crash, every coarse accent – makes her want to put her hands over her ears. There are beeps like bullets of noise assailing her, announcements like klaxons breaking a fitful sleep – and the hospital smells rancid, like an abandoned refrigerator.

Catherine staggers slowly along the corridor, squeezing Annie's hand. It's a trap. She has to escape this place, whatever happens she has to leave.

The world – by which I mean everything we experience as reality – is not just presented to us like a movie. The world is not separate from us. We're not in the audience.

Sarah's hospital and Catherine's hospital are different places. It would be ridiculous to say that they are not.

Who is the Real Patient?

Who is Catherine?

Catherine is at home now. Annie has left her alone, with tea and chocolates and a promise to call this evening. Catherine is feeling upset and confused. She has an illness. She is going to forget more and more. So she sits and concentrates and tries to remember the past.

She was so happy at school – a star. Head girl in the end, before university. She got distracted there, she remembers, but she can't exactly recall why? Was it a boy? A love? An unexpected passion? She's not sure.

A job. A writer – a reporter. A house with a picket fence. Family meals. A daughter: Annie. Yes, Annie. And a son.

Catherine thumps the arm of her chair. Tears well. She can see her son in her mind but for God's sake she can't remember his name. Johnny? Jimmy? James? She holds her head in her brown-flecked hands.

The phone rings. She doesn't answer.

Elsewhere, Annie is talking to her father, Peter. She's breaking the bad news about Catherine.

> There's not much we can do Dad. We just have to keep talking to her. Talking about her favourite things, what she loved to do.
>
> She comes and goes at the moment. Sometimes she seems fine then she goes vacant. It's scary. It's like I'm losing my Mum and friend before my eyes. It's like she's leaking out of her body…

Annie tries to hold back sobs. Peter is unsympathetic.

> I know she's your mother Annie, and I feel for you, but you don't see her like I do. She was awful to me when we were married. Spiteful. Vindictive. Self-centred. All she seemed to care about was herself … To be honest, if that part of her is disappearing then I won't mourn it.

'How can you say that?' Annie yells at him.

Maybe you should think of the reasons why she ended up not liking you. Maybe you should look at yourself? Mum's a good person. Kind, loving, naïve … She'd help anyone in need – she helped you remember, when she didn't need to and when you didn't deserve it. I don't want to lose her kindness. I wish we could save her, Dad …

Who is Sarah?

The next day Sarah's in a team meeting. It's her first day as a nurse manager. She's feeling proud and enthusiastic.

The team is looking at the hospital budget, looking to save money but keep quality at the same time. They are considering staffing levels, which are a little high compared to the national average.

Sarah is flicking through the budget sheets, looking for places where cost reductions can be achieved. She puts her finger on geriatric care, thinking of all the elderly people who contribute little or nothing to the economy, and never will again. She thinks of senile patients – they scare her actually – she doesn't understand them. Where are they? What's the point of living without memory? How is that living at all?

She briefly remembers an old lady yesterday, she bumped into her as she was leaving the doctor's office. Another one bites the dust, she thought. It won't be long until that one's in long stay, god knows for how long. But why? If she forgets then how does it matter where she is?

Sarah looks up.

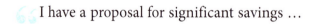
I have a proposal for significant savings …

Who is the Real Patient?

Is there just one Catherine, or many? It seems obvious that there are many – there's Catherine's view of herself and her life. There's Annie's view. There's Peter's view. There's Sarah's view. Does it really make any sense to say there is one correct view? Or is the patient a complex, ever-changing reality: a human kaleidoscope?

If we – as carers – take only one perspective of the patient as real, then we're accepting a delusion – a passing mirage – as a truth.

Appearance, Reality and the Values Delusion

The reason most people are deluded about values is that we do not appreciate that we continually create realities, as we combine the external world with our reactions to it. We're so used to a deluge of information that we think we don't matter. We think the reality we see would exist even if we didn't, so accustomed have we become to thinking we receive the world passively, like empty buckets. But we are mistaken.

For example, take this situation. You can respond to it on the Values Exchange if you like.

STOP & THINK ELEVEN: MARMADUKE'S SAD DEMISE

Josephine is a frail elderly lady who is being treated for pneumonia in the hospital where you work as a nurse. She is making a recovery and has a good prognosis.

However, she seems very anxious and keeps asking about her cat, who has been left in the care of the neighbours.

You enquire with the neighbours about the cat – Marmaduke – and sadly they tell you that he was run over and killed this morning. They beg you not to tell Josephine about this because they fear it will set her back and make her not want to recover. They think the shock might be too much for her in her condition, and you know that bad news can cause relapses for physical problems like pneumonia.

You go back to the ward unsure what to do for the best. Josephine calls you over and asks you directly, 'Please nurse, do you know how Marmaduke is?'

What should you do?

It is proposed that you tell Josephine about her cat.

Add your response on the Values Exchange: http://thoughtful.vxcommunity.com/Issue/think-stop-eleven-marmaduke-s-sad-demise/19544

According to the **Official View**, if you are wearing the 'I'm an honest person' t-shirt, like everyone else who's wearing it, you will know what to do. All the honest people will share the same value and do the same thing. But, as we've seen, this doesn't – indeed it cannot – actually happen.

This point should be clear enough by now, but even this is not fundamental.

The fundamental point is that if you are Josephine's carer, needing to decide what to do for the best, your experience of reality, in the moment where she is asking you about Marmaduke, is a unique relationship created by your physical abilities and reactions, your history, your memories, your training, your preferences at that point, your fondness for your own cat – everything that makes you who you are – combined with everything that makes the external world what it is – Josephine's eyes, her voice, the hospital smells, how much time you have, whether anyone else is with you – simply everything. Reality for you – in this slice of time – is the impossibly complex relationship between you and the external influences on you.

This does not mean that you will therefore decide randomly, or that you can go either way just as readily – you will have your preferences, as a part of the mix that creates your decision. But it does mean that the idea that you are guided by your values alone is obviously wrong.

We Mix Ourselves with Everything Around Us

If the reality we experience is always a relationship between the data we receive and how we react to it, then values simply cannot be as they are on the **Official View**.

Values cannot exist out of context. The only time we can be sure we have a value is when we are doing something. It's meaningless to say 'I have this value' in the abstract. Values come into being when we react to what's happening around us.

Adding a standard label – like 'honesty' or 'compassion' – to a fleeting relationship between what's happening and what you are doing about it, obscures its uniqueness. Of course, we all have abiding preferences, and we are predictable to an extent, but each time we decide we create a new reality, with no guarantee of consistency.

Here is another example that you can investigate yourself on the Values Exchange. You can respond to the issue in your own way, but it is at least as instructive to look at and think about others' responses, and the reasons why they responded as they did.

So long as you submit a response yourself on the Values Exchange you will have access to everyone else's ideas.

STOP & THINK TWELVE: BLURRED BOUNDARY?

Jimmy, a 25-year-old man who suffers with Bipolar Disorder, has been admitted to the unit voluntarily, following increasing depression and suicidal thoughts of late. Over the previous few weeks Jimmy has become very withdrawn and has been isolating himself from his family and friends.

As one of Jimmy's health care workers, you feel it is imperative that you are able to build a therapeutic alliance with him, in order to ascertain trust and rapport which will assist in enabling Jimmy to communicate openly with you and to enable you to establish, with the team, his suicidal risk.

Jimmy smokes heavily, and although there is a no-smoking policy in operation within the Trust, Jimmy frequently visits the 'square' outside, which sits within the unit, to have a cigarette.

On this particular morning Jimmy is restless and when you enquire as to what the problem is, he says he has no cigarettes. You are a smoker, and in your quest to get close to Jimmy, and get to know him, you offer him one of yours and ask him if he would like to share a cigarette with you in the square.

Jimmy agrees to sit and have a cigarette with you outside.

It is proposed that despite policy you continue to step outside with Jimmy to share a cigarette with him.

(Case prepared by Vanessa Peutherer, VX Learning Facilitator)

Here is one actual comment (unedited) from Jenny (this isn't her real name):

> **Jenny: Disagreed** 'I dont smoke dont understand it ..makes you ill, i would not encourage any smoking ,smoke free for me sorry you smoker's.'

Here's an alternative comment and decision (again unedited and unidentified):

> **Josie: Agreed** because – Although my head tells me this is wrong my heart tells me otherwise. I feel it would be good to try and connect with jimmy and build up a trust and understanding with him so he will benefit in the long run, as long as this dosnt become a

regular habit and he knows that, i dont see any harm im sure we have all been led by our hearts instead of our heads at some time.

I use these examples because they give a sense of the reality of our perceptions of each other and the naïvety of assuming that we decide according to solid, fixed values.

The way Jenny sees the client creates a different reality from that forged by Josie, who sees the client in another light. Despite what commonsense begs us to believe, there is not just one client whom everyone is able to understand in the same way, rather there are many realities of that person, which depend on what the person is, does and says and how you react to that.

This is a mind-boggling insight.

It's impossible for any of us to know other people exactly as they are. It's impossible for any of us to know ourselves as we really are. The 'really are' aspects of people are forever hidden behind our veils of perception.

However, throughout this book there are several techniques we can use to get closer.

Jenny's brief comment is particularly interesting, not because of its insight but because it is real. Jenny doesn't like smoking so she won't support the patient.

Yes, it is a value-judgement. She says, 'I don't like smoking so I'm not going to sit with him.' Apparently simple enough, but underlying this judgement there's a whole history – which we are unlikely ever to know and which is at least partly hidden from Jenny too. It is these underlying influences – many of them subtle: risk to job? Risk of looking bad to others? Ex-smoker in denial? Dislike of Jimmy? Fondness of Jimmy? Belief that smokers are weak? It's this, not lists of 'Big Values' or official codes, that create our decisions.

Jenny looks at Jimmy and creates one reality, which is different from the reality created by Josie. One client, two carers, two different versions of the client. Whether to support Jimmy's smoking or not is not to do with values in any conventional sense. It is to do with impressions, passing interactions, feelings, instincts, indoctrination, conditioned reflexes, biology – it's very much more raw than most of us are prepared even to contemplate.

SUMMARY OF CHAPTER 3

1. There is no doubt that the way things appear to we human beings is not the way things really are. It's simply not possible for us to access pure, unadulterated reality. Everything we receive from the world outside us is filtered by our senses, our beliefs, our education, our era, our sciences, our technologies. No-one sees exactly the same world, because no-one is the same as anyone else.
2. The reality we experience is created by relationships. It is a result of the relationship between the data we receive and our own interpretation of it – and this interpretation is affected by every part of us: physical, psychological, emotional, historical, political, and so on.
3. This is a vital insight for health carers of all kinds. Once you understand that reality is a relationship, and therefore different for everyone, you are able to explore rich possibilities, and you are constantly aware that there is so much more behind whatever label is currently stuck on a patient. For example, if you think reality is truly only what you personally think it is, you may conclude that a person who is petrified to receive an injection is obviously 'over-anxious'. But if you ask instead, 'how can it be that this person is so frightened?', 'what is it in her perception of the needle that makes the reality of the needle for her so intimidating?' then while you may never know for sure you will at least be open to seeing the world closer to the way she does, rather than projecting your view of the needle – and of her – on to her.
4. Hospitals and patients will appear one way to us, but will appear differently to other people. What may be a routine procedure to us may be terrifying to a patient, because their reality will be different from ours, shaped as it is by so many personal factors and past experiences. A central health care task is to try to understand as much as possible about other people's realities, and their causes.

SUMMARY OF THE BOOK SO FAR

It's worth pausing for a moment to take stock. In a way what I am saying in this book is very simple, but it's not intuitive, so here's the bones of it so far.

1. Iggy – the black labrador – sees the world in an entirely different way from the way humans see the world.
2. We assume that the way we see the world is superior to Iggy's, but this is just hubris.
3. There can be no doubt that an external world exists independent of human beings. However, the human way of seeing things is just one way to view reality.
4. We assume we all see the same world.

(Continued)

(Continued)

5. But reality is not a given, it's an experience. In 'philosophy-speak', reality is continually created by a relationship between external data received by our senses, and our interpretation of the data we receive.
6. In order for us to communicate when we all have different perspectives, we need labels (which are based on a shared language and shared meanings).
7. These labels give us the power to categorise reality, to shape it because we can understand it up to a point, and to talk meaningfully with each other. In one way our labels free and empower us.
8. However, we often confuse our labels for reality itself. For example, we use values as labels and immediately conclude that therefore values truly exist as simple, separate aspects of reality. But this is delusion.
9. We are addicted to our labels. We find it very hard – and often impossible – to peel them away.
10. Like focussing a camera using 'depth of field' – as we home in on what we have labelled, the rest of reality (the rest of the meadow) blurs.
11. Because we label distinct parts of our meadows we learn to think of reality in separate packets, rather than a connected whole.
12. Our labels also inhibit us. They may give us a certain kind of insight – but used thoughtlessly they blind us to everything else that might matter.
13. In one way we are freer than Iggy – we have more power, thanks to the technologies and social connections our labelling has helped us build. In another way Iggy is freer than us because – apart from his instincts – he has no preconceptions, and he is not affected by any labels which tell him how to think and what to do. Iggy's perceptions are not polluted by labels.

You can look at the meadow as a botanist or a housing developer or as a dog and you will not see the same meadow. Yet we all assume that the meadow we see is the same meadow everyone else sees.

Our journey in the next chapter will show, with many practical examples, just how mistaken we are.

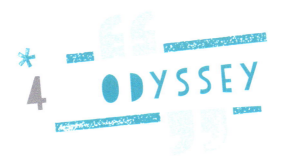

We interpret reality in our own ways, in every facet of our lives. Once our version of reality becomes comfortable to us we get complacent, satisfied with the truth we've made up. Very often, we get so content we stop thinking altogether.

Though this book is mostly for health workers of all kinds, it's important to be aware that no aspect of life is immune to our acquired habit of thoughtlessness. Consequently, this chapter embarks on a brief odyssey across an apparently random set of subjects, to show how easy it is to become intellectually numb. It also explains, by example, how simple methods of thought and awareness can be used to powerful effect – no matter what area of life you are considering.

Risk is the perfect place to start, since risk is so often the biggest label on the packet.

Risk

Risks are generally regarded as isolated elements in life. To us risks are like banana skins on pavements – hazards to be swept up before someone gets hurt. Or they're like meteors coming at us out of the sky: huge, separate extra-terrestrial boulders to be shot down and destroyed, like aliens in a video game.

To the establishment mind, risks are spikey little problems we must eliminate if we're to enjoy smooth, trouble-free lives. But there's a strange phenomenon – the more we try to eradicate risk the more risks there seem to be. It's like the toddlers' toy with plastic clowns hiding in holes on a game board. Whenever a clown pops up the child's supposed to hit him back down with a hammer, yet this merely causes another clown to pop out from another hole, endlessly.

The problem here – as you may have guessed – is seeing risks as separate when it makes no sense to do so.

The Strange Case of the Dangerous Flowers

The UK newspaper, the *Daily Mail*, recently highlighted a bizarre but far from unusual 'health care risk', leading with the headline:

> FLOWERS BAN AT 9 IN 10 HOSPITALS: INCREASING NUMBERS INTRODUCE RULES AFTER CONCERNS BLOOMS SPREAD GERMS AND CREATE EXTRA WORK FOR NURSES
>
> A splash of colour in an otherwise dreary hospital ward can brighten up even the most difficult of days.
>
> But according to a survey, nine out of ten NHS hospitals do not allow patients to have fresh flowers by their bed – despite three out of four people opposing a ban.
>
> Increasing numbers of hospitals have introduced the rules to address concerns about spreading germs, aggravating allergies and creating extra work for nurses.
>
> However, the poll of 3,700 Britons discovered that around 90 per cent said flowers can dramatically improve someone's mood when they are unwell, and almost half thought they would speed up recovery. Just over three-quarters of people surveyed disagreed with banning the gifts.'
>
> There's no official ruling from the Department of Health on whether flowers should be allowed in wards.

Craft supplier Country Baskets, who conducted the poll said 'we appreciate the concerns around taking flowers on to wards. But there are real, proven benefits to giving flowers to people who are unwell.' And psychologist Emma Kenny pointed to evidence that 'many studies … show the psychological impact that flowers can have on a person's recovery or general well-being …' (73). Nevertheless, despite the many positives associated with flowers, according to the poll of 105 hospitals there was a fresh flower ban in 97 of them, with the rest discouraging visitors from bringing bouquets.

Apart from the fact that there's no clear evidence of any risk caused by having flowers on wards (74), there's a much deeper consideration here. The case of the dangerous flowers perfectly illustrates the mistake of seeing the world in packets.

Someone or other – maybe a few people, it's unlikely to be more – looked at flowers in hospitals and identified them as 'a risk' – with the emphasis on 'a'. According to these 'risk detectives', flowers on wards are a self-contained problem which, once prevented, will remove a single risk. Get rid of the flowers – another risk bites the dust. End of story.

But like any other perceived problem, not only is it we who say whether and to what extent something is a risk, but if you get rid of one risk you never do so without consequences. The world is not made up of disconnected elements – it's a rich and deeply inter-related tapestry where affecting one thread is bound to affect other threads, just like the butterfly effect (75). Alternatively, you might think of reality as an intricate curry, where if you remove one ingredient you will inevitably change the entire dish.

What's the Risk of Preventing this Risk?

Because we live in a connected world – if you ban flowers you may stop one perceived risk but you're bound to create new ones. Banning 'dangerous flowers', for example, will at the very least cause:

- A less beautiful environment: a ward full of flowers is much prettier than one without them.
- Less happy patients, especially those who love flowers and gardens.
- Reduced psychological well-being and longer recovery times.
- Reduced patient choice and autonomy: if I'm prevented from having flowers at my bedside I am likely to feel disempowered and trapped.
- Conflict between staff and patients/visitors who want to bring in flowers: if I'm visiting my friend in hospital with a bouquet of flowers and I'm prevented from delivering them, not only will I feel frustrated and sad, but I might well end up arguing with the staff member who has to implement the ban, whether it's her choice or not.

- An environment in which the whole notion of risk is inflated beyond what can possibly be considered sensible.
- An environment where patients become increasingly scared and fearful about all the risks they hear about.
- Unnecessary anxiety amongst patients and relatives about having flowers at home when they're sick.
- Demotivation amongst staff who have not been involved in this decision (obviously not everyone agrees with the flower ban, which is an imposed decision – and imposing decisions on people itself brings many risks).
- A ripple effect – or slippery slope – where further quite normal and safe situations and practices fall under the official gaze, as the 'risk bar' is subtly lowered further and further (allowing patients to have books for example could be seen as an infection risk, or possibly an injury hazard, if they are large and heavy books).

Part of the risk phobia problem is lack of institutional imagination, and lack of power – or guts – in employees afraid of the consequences to them as individuals. As soon as someone identifies a perceived risk everyone panics.

> We have to take this seriously. What if it actually happens and we didn't do anything about it?
>
> Something has to be done. We have to manage this situation. We can't keep the lid on this. Let's make it official so everyone can see we are managing risk effectively.

A Simple Question

Preventing one risk sets off a cascade of further risks, but this is rarely understood. As a cure I suggest the simplest of questions. Whenever it occurs to someone to prevent a risk they should ask:

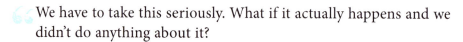

What's the risk of preventing this risk?

There will always be further risks. It's just the way things are.

As Allen Buchanan writes:

> Eliminating risk isn't possible. Life isn't like that. But even if it were possible, eliminating risk would be a mistake, because the costs of doing this would be too high …
>
> Here's an example. Suppose we can achieve a 10 per cent reduction of serious injury in a car crash for every additional one eighth inch of steel we add to the body of a car. If we add enough to make the doors as thick as the hull of an Abrams tank, nobody will die in a car crash … But beyond a certain point, an additional increment of risk reduction … isn't worth it. The car becomes unaffordable and the cost of gas for such a heavy vehicle becomes prohibitive. (76)

The packet trap is an enormous hindrance to us. We are deeply confused by it. Under its spell all our supposedly bright ideas and efforts are repeatedly in vain.

As Michael Power comments:

> Risk talk and risk management practices, rather like auditing in the 1990s, embody the fundamentally contradictory nature of organisational and political life. On the one hand there is a functional and political need to maintain myths of control and manageability, because this is what various interested constituencies and stakeholders seem to demand. Risks must be made auditable and governable.
>
> On the other hand, there is a consistent stream of failures, scandals and disasters which challenge and threaten organisations, suggesting a world which is out of control and where failure may be endemic, and in which the organisational interdependencies are so intricate that no single locus of control has a grasp of them. (77)

A clown pops up from the hole. Someone hits him. Immediately a new clown – sometimes several new clowns – pop out of other holes.

If you feel like reflecting further, consider the following issue. As always, you can think independently, discuss with friends and colleagues, debate in class if you have one or you can go to the Values Exchange to share your views with others, and then access the continually growing reports.

STOP & THINK THIRTEEN: ACTIONS SPEAK LOUDER THAN WORDS?

Bill is a 78-year-old man, widowed six months ago. Bill is in the post-op recovery stage following a total hip replacement three days previously. Apart from some mild Atrial Fibrillation, Arthritis and Reactive Depression (since the sudden death of his wife, Edith) Bill is considered to be reasonably fit and well. No complications for discharge are anticipated at this time.

As a Health Care Support Worker on the Unit, you've noticed that Bill appears to be more withdrawn since his operation and frequently keeps his door shut. You knock and enter and find Bill sat in his chair, beside his bed, playing cards on the table in front of him. As the ward is quiet, you ask Bill if he would like to partner you in a few games of Pontoon. Bill smiles and accepts and gestures for you pull up the chair opposite him.

Whilst playing, Bill starts to talk of how he always played cards with his wife daily. Suddenly his eyes fill up and he begins to cry. You move the table away from in front of him and move from your chair. In an attempt to get closer to Bill, you sit on the bed next to his chair and hold his outstretched hand.

A few moments later the Staff Nurse walks past the door, which is still ajar. She deliberately raises her voice, ordering you to 'get off the bed'.

You are aware that in order to prevent the risk of cross infection, it's Trust Infection Control Policy for staff to refrain from sitting on patients' beds, but you are more concerned about Bill's immediate needs. The only other place to sit, due to lack of space, is in the chair opposite and further away from Bill, as there's no room to move the chair adjacent to him.

Bill looks worried and tells you, 'You should go, I don't want you to get into trouble.'
What's the risk here?
What's the compassionate thing to do here?
It is proposed that you continue to talk with Bill, sitting on the bed.

(Case prepared by Vanessa Peutherer, VX Learning Facilitator)

 Add your response on the Values Exchange: http://thoughtful.vxcommunity.com/Issue/think-stop-thirteen-actions-speak-louder-than-words/21946

In the end, it's all rather silly:

> Concerning the prohibition in some UK hospitals against visitors, nurses or doctors being allowed to sit on a patient's bed … (patients) could make an informed choice – between keeping all humans at a safe distance at least an arm's length away or allowing staff and visitors to sit on their bed, shedding the odd skin flake and bacteria, but with

the intangible benefit of conveying a sense of intimacy and kindness. I know what I would choose … Banning bed sitting will do nothing to reduce infection levels but will reduce the ability of health professionals and loved ones to bring healing and comfort to patients. (78)

Apart from the fact that not being allowed to sit on patients' beds is in total opposition to the NHS Constitution which, you may remember, says 'NHS services must reflect, and should be coordinated around and tailored to, the needs and preferences of patients, their families and their carers …', the ramifications of the staff nurse's actions are enormous. Her instruction to you (in the **STOP & THINK** above) is not in a packet. It's part of the flow of life, not separate from it. Bill gets sadder. You get resentful. Bill goes off his food, and gets weaker. You start to wonder if the hospital is really the place for you. You start to think what else you might be doing … a butterfly flaps its wings and a chain reaction ensues.

School

We are deluded one way or another from the moment we're born – but once we get to school things really ramp up. Many of our delusions begin there because schools have *labelmania*. Schools teach children about goblins, not the meadow.

Enter pretty much any school anywhere in the world and you'll experience a barrage of labels: visitors' labels at the reception desk, clocks on the wall, timetables split into separate periods of time for separate subjects, lockers with student names on, every room labelled on the outside, and inside every wall plastered with information: things to remember, facts and figures, codes of behaviour, honours boards, gold stars, student work neatly labelled with student name and age. You'll find store rooms for files with labels on, form rooms, student leaders, prefects, head boys and girls, each with deputies – an orderly world exquisitely divided into bite size pieces. Attend school prize-giving events and labelmania turns gale force. Student after student winning category after category: excellence in maths, a cup in Spanish, best in year, overall Dux – and everyone in a uniform, just in case there's any doubt you could be anywhere else but a school claiming to support creativity and independence in young people.

Of course, many students enjoy school, have positive experiences and even learn there. And there's no doubt there are good teachers, sensitive not only to the needs of their students but also to the artificial and potentially damaging environment in which they work. That said, there's even less doubt that schools are the puppet-masters of delusion.

To most of us, school seems normal. We expect children to start aged five or earlier, we expect them to be tested, we expect them to be in competition with one another, we understand there are some 'must do well in' subjects (like maths) and others that are optional (like dance), we expect teachers to make sure classes are orderly and we generally believe that 'bad behaviour' will be punished for the good of the offender, for the good of others, and for the reputation of the school.

Yet viewed another way, contemporary schooling is an extraordinary act of socially sanctioned delusion – offering its own, made-up, classifications as a natural truth.

Undeniably, a primary purpose of the school system is to force young people to conform to its rules, systems, goals and values. It's hard to find a school that does not openly admit to this in its official materials – prospectuses, curricula, missions, principals' welcomes and so on. This might just be OK were schools to be fair, effective and not compulsory, but just consider what happens to students who don't like school, are not interested in school and its random subjects or who happen not to be very good at passing the tests associated with them. Students who fall into this category are labelled as failures, drop outs, lazy, stupid – take your pick from any number of derogatory titles.

As Ivan Illich observed:

> Most learning is not the result of instruction. It is rather the result of unhampered participation in a meaningful setting. Most people learn best by being 'with it', yet school makes them identify their personal, cognitive growth with elaborate planning and manipulation … Schools are designed on the assumption that there is a secret to everything in life; that the quality of life depends on knowing that secret; that secrets can be known only in orderly successions; and that only teachers can properly reveal these secrets. An individual with a schooled mind conceives of the world as a pyramid of classified packages accessible only to those who carry the proper tags. (79)

Illich again:

> A second major illusion on which the school system rests is that most learning is the result of teaching ... Teaching, it is true, may contribute to certain kinds of learning under certain circumstances. But most people acquire most of their knowledge outside school, and in school only in so far as school, in a few rich countries, has become their place of confinement during an increasing part of their lives. (79)

It's not just confinement. It's brainwashing too. As an extreme example (or is it?) some schools in Israel proudly indoctrinate children as an essential aspect of what they do – including having teachers in kindergarten in military uniform. Palestinians (the enemy) are depicted not with openness and curiosity toward another culture – but as goblins (either terrorists or primitive farmers) with barbaric histories and little human similarity to the apparently more civilised Israelis. Just as my boyhood comic books – *The Victor*, *The Hotspur* and so on – ruthlessly propagandised the evil Hun (80).

Ken Robinson has become famous for his humorous and damning criticism of schools' fixation with not only labels, but a very specifically organised sets of labels. Sir Robinson asks: why are some subjects regarded as premier and others optional?

He argues that the whole Western education system is based on traditional academic ability, and simply refuses to cater for students who have other talents:

> If you think of it, the whole system of public education around the world is a protracted process of university entrance. And the consequence is that many highly-talented, brilliant, creative people think they're not, because the thing they were good at at [sic] school wasn't valued, or was actually stigmatized. (81)

Not only is a galaxy of knowledge and inquiry divided into tiny packets in school, some of the packets are rated as more important than others. Maths and English are seen as essential while Art and Dance are optional because, Robinson says, the education system was designed to meet the needs of industrialisation – teaching essential work skills – not the needs of creative children (82).

Other commentators, such as the artist Suli, make similar points in less conventional ways, in raps explaining that education is about inspiring minds rather than passing exams, and that education can be about anything, not just some official list of detached, recommended 'top subjects'. Suli tells us he once saw David Beckham take a free kick, the ball soared in one direction then swerved in another, the goalkeeper froze shocked by the ball apparently disobeying the laws of physics, before the goal was scored and the crowd erupted. Thinking of Beckham's footballing skills, Suli concludes, quite rightly, that there is more than one way to be an educated man (83).

Not every school system is deluded. Finnish schooling, for example, offers a positive model of anti-separatist education. Impressively, in 2015 the Finns decided not to teach by separate subjects any more, but to have students investigate topics in which lots of different skills and knowledge need to come together to be effective. The Finns call this 'phenomenon teaching' – for instance, a teenager studying a vocational course might take 'cafeteria services' lessons, which may include elements of maths, languages (to help serve foreign customers), writing skills and communication skills. More academic pupils might be taught cross-subject topics, like 'what is the European Union and why does it exist?' which would, for example, combine elements of economics, history, languages and geography (84).

Luck

Frano Selak has been dubbed 'the world's luckiest man'. According to the UK newspaper *Daily Telegraph*, the 87-year-old (2016) music teacher 'cheated death' seven times before winning a million dollars in the Croatian lottery. The newspaper tells a good story. Apparently, Frano had his first escape in 1962 when a train he was travelling on from Sarajevo to Dubrovnik jumped the rails and plunged into an icy river. Seventeen people drowned and he barely made it to the riverbank after suffering from hypothermia, shock, bruises and a broken arm.

A year later, he was thrown out of a plane on his first and only flight when a door flew open. This time 19 people died but he was thrown clear of the crash and landed in a haystack.

Then in 1966, a bus he was on skidded into a river, drowning four. He swam to safety with just cuts and bruises.

Accident number four came in 1970 when his car caught fire as he drove along a motorway and he fled with seconds to spare before the fuel tank exploded.

Three years later, he lost most of his hair when a faulty fuel pump spewed petrol over the hot engine of his car and blew flames through the air vents.

Then in 1995 came his sixth accident when he was knocked down by a bus in Zagreb but walked away with minor injuries.

The following year, he was driving in the mountains when he turned a corner to see a UN truck coming straight for him.

His Skoda careered through a crash barrier and over the 300ft precipice. But he leapt clear at the last moment and sat in a tree as he watched his car hit the bottom and explode.

He then won £600,000 with his first ever lottery ticket and celebrated his fifth marriage saying, 'I guess all the earlier marriages were disasters too.' (85)

Rather charmingly, Mr Selak gave away his fortune, claiming that all he needed was the love of his fifth wife, Katrina. Frano is quoted as saying, '… when she arrived I knew then that I really did have a charmed, blessed life …' Even more refreshing, the 'luckiest man alive' refuses to go along with the media hype. He reckons he 'never thought I was lucky to survive all my brushes with death. I thought I was unlucky to be in them in the first place.'

By contrast, Listverse.com carries an upsetting (or amusing – dependent on your propensity to *Schadenfreude*) list of what it calls 'the 9 unluckiest people ever' (86). The list includes the only man of a village of 70 households not to have signed up for a collective lottery ticket worth many millions; the American woman who lost five houses to five hurricanes; 'Calamity' John Lyne, a UK citizen who has suffered 16 major accidents including lightning strikes, a rock fall in a mine and three car crashes (apparently, as a teen, after breaking his arm falling from a tree, John went to hospital for treatment. On the way home from hospital the bus he was travelling on crashed, causing him to break the same arm in a different place); and Tsutomu Yamagochi who was the only officially recognised person to endure both the Hiroshima and Nagasaki atomic bomb blasts at the end of World War II (87).

While these tales may seem a humorous distraction, there's a more serious point here: 'luck' is a superstition not a fact, but we are so used to thinking it exists that we forget that luck doesn't actually occur in nature, rather it's just in our heads and our mythology.

It's very tempting to label people – and ourselves – as lucky or unlucky, and hardly any of us fail to hope for more luck ourselves and to wish it on others. But just because an idea is commonplace and seemingly widely understood by everyone, it does not follow that it's real. 'Luck' exists only in so far as we invoke the idea to explain what would otherwise seem arbitrary – random, meaningless events occurring 'in the raw', for no reason whatsoever. Because we are physically and mentally built to find and recognise patterns, and to ascribe meaning to those patterns, we're more comfortable with labels like 'luck' or 'karma' or 'fortune' than 'chance' or 'it just happened' – but what exactly is luck? How and where does it exist? How is it that some people are lucky and others are not? As far as anyone knows there is no mechanism for luck, no magic spell to create it and no method for making oneself luckier. Instead, there is nature in the raw and our attempt to make it fit with a reassuring way of looking at and coping with it.

Frano Selak is 'the world's luckiest man' only if we say he is.

'Luck' is simply one more way in which we try to make sense of the chaos that surrounds us. Accepting this – accepting that luck is merely a means by which we cushion ourselves against a pointless universe – is a good thing because it frees us from delusion, if only a little. If we believe in luck then we will ascribe a particular, limited meaning to events and situations. But if we understand that luck is a label, then we are able to use the label if we want – and perhaps talk to patients about their luck if that is one of their means of coping – and we can also talk about reality without that label. For example, patients often ask 'why me?' – 'why did I get cancer?' – 'why did this happen to me and not to my friends?' Free of the delusion you can talk about luck if you think it might help, and you can also talk about a world where there is no luck and where things 'just happen', for no meaningful reason: a world not set for or against you – a world that doesn't care, a world of pitiless indifference to our goals and our suffering.

The challenge for you as a health worker is to decide what sort of conversation will be most liberating for the patient. And you have more options the more delusions you have overcome.

Disability

Disabled or a Person with Disabilities?

One very clear example of how labels powerfully and instantly shape our perceptions is our labelling of ourselves and other people. We're not content – possibly we're unable – simply to see other human individuals just as people, rather we're driven to select certain aspects of them above others: mother, singer, ethicist, drummer, terminal patient, schizophrenic, winner, loser. In other words, we're all journalists of our own perceptions, wrapping each other up in parcels we can handle, just like mediocre news pundits who can't see past the headlines.

So how do we label a man in a wheelchair or a woman who finds it hard to read and write because she doesn't find learning easy. What labels should we stick on them? There are – of course – a lot to choose from.

Whatever label we choose, we are bound to create a diminished reality as we do so. This has been clear forever to 'disabled people' – see how impossible it is for us not to use labels? Even apparently positive labels diminish. Rob Crossan – an albino man – says:

> I tend to react rather badly whenever people do call me "brave" for being able to catch a bus, write a feature or order a kebab, despite my albinism. Because I simply do not deserve the praise. And not only is it deeply patronising to congratulate me for simply living my life, it also grates because I know that being called "inspiring" by an able-bodied person is merely their way of projecting the fact that, until they met me, the last time they had an emotional connection with a disabled person was when they saw one cross the finish line in Stratford a couple of years ago. (88)

Most people, most of the time, are happy to be called 'inspiring'. But not if in so labelling them their real self is obscured.

Whatever label we use to describe 'a disabled person' not only 'badges' that person as 'limited' or 'needy' or 'less capable' or 'inspiring' or 'brave' and so on, but it causes an entirely false divide between 'disabled' people and the rest of us. Any label we choose to use that says 'this set of abilities' is less desirable than another set of abilities is pasted onto reality by us, it is not reality itself.

All there is – the other side of our labelling – is a human world with billions of people, all with different abilities. It is we who decide to make positive or negative judgements about these abilities, and these people. We are all disabled in most ways, but while we think there is a category called 'disabled people' and another category called 'non-disabled people' we remain blind to this otherwise completely obvious fact. I can't play soccer any more – it hurts my joints too much – so in this regard I am, if I want to label myself, disabled. If you compare me with Ronaldo then I am most definitely in need of 'special assistance', since I am in a totally different category from the Portuguese soccer player. But I can swim and cycle well so – compared to most people I am not disabled in these areas, though I am in comparison to the winner of the Tour de France or the 100 metre sprint at the Olympics. Compared to Stephen Hawkins there is hardly any way in which I might be considered physically disabled, but as far as my skills in Physics are concerned I have hardly any ability at all – I could very plausibly define myself – or be defined by others (a school or a university for example) as disabled or a 'special needs' candidate in Physics.

It's all so arbitrary. We are all disabled in most areas of life and we all have at least some abilities in other areas. All of us are in many ways a desert and in many ways a meadow, even people with apparently 'profound disabilities', like Helen Keller who was blind, deaf and mute but nevertheless became an internationally renowned educator and social activist (89).

Rights

There are many commissions and institutions that concern themselves with 'human rights'. These institutions not only make lists of human rights and wrap them up as truths, but they collude and confer with one another to lend weight and credibility to their declarations. Not all their rights are consistent with each other, but that doesn't seem to matter since everybody intuitively knows what human rights are, don't they?

In fact, any claim to a natural right is just that – a claim not a truth. Nature itself does not contain goodness, badness or human rights – just processes, objects, events – raw data, which we process and make of it what we will:

> …there is nothing either good or bad, but thinking makes it so. To me it is a prison. (90)

There's reality in the raw – nature as it would be without our interpretation of it – and then there are human institutions – in this case with a desire to claim that human rights are natural, factual and would exist 'in the raw', even if we had no words. But human rights do not exist 'in the raw' – they are nowhere to be found until we say they exist.

One very obvious problem with having a plethora of human rights is that they can conflict both in theory and practice, which of course means that legislators, judges and governments pick the rights they want, and discard the ones they don't. It's up to us, for our own reasons, to say one right is more important than another: for example, the right to own as much property as you like – over another right – the right to income equality. Such prioritising is not natural – it simply our choosing and our labelling.

As Eric Posner – an American law professor – writes in the UK newspaper *The Guardian*:

> The Americans argued that human rights consisted of political rights – the rights to vote, to speak freely, not to be arbitrarily detained, to practise a religion of one's own choice, and so on … The Soviets argued that human rights consisted of social or economic rights – the rights to work, to health care, and to education … the result was that negotiations to convert the universal declaration (of Human Rights) into a binding treaty were split into two tracks … (then, after 18 years) … the United Nations adopted a political rights treaty and an economic rights treaty (rather than a unified one). (91)

Or, as Jeremy Bentham put it, rather more directly,

> rights is the child of law, from real law come real rights; but from imaginary laws, from "law of nature" come imaginary rights … Natural rights is … nonsense upon stilts. (92)

Rights are easily dispensed with when it suits. For example, in order to implement what is known as 'the Northern Territory Intervention', in 2007 the Australian government chose to suspend the Racial Discrimination Act, so removing any legal protections Aboriginal and Torres Strait Island People in the Northern Territory had against racial discrimination. White people were not affected by the Northern Territory Intervention.

Black people's legal rights were removed as the result of a report on child abuse in order to protect women and children through a range of measures including the restriction of alcohol (Aboriginals were simply not allowed to buy it or have it), more police in communities and the quarantining of welfare payments (Aboriginals could only spend the money on approved items). Any appeal from Aboriginal people to their supposedly deeper 'natural rights' – for example the right to self-determination and the right to have their stolen lands back – fell on deaf white ears (93).

The News

News media perfectly exemplify the packet trap. Rolf Dobelli – a Swiss author and businessman – compares the news we are currently spoon-fed to sugar for the body:

> News is easy to digest. The media feeds us small bites of trivial matter, tidbits [sic] that don't require thinking … we can swallow limitless quantities of news flashes, like bright colored candies for the mind. (94)

To test out his belief that modern news delivery is toxic, Dobelli went without consuming any news for a year – leading, he says, to less disruption, more time, less anxiety, deeper thinking and more insights. This really should not surprise us – if we allow news-media to make sense of the world for us, and if their way of making sense for us is to throw random stories, facts, anecdotes and asides at us – in an incoherent jumble – we should hardly be surprised that we switch off and find our minds increasingly numb.

Dobelli argues that the way news-media habitually pick on certain topics and not others creates a completely wrong map of risk in our heads – totally misrepresenting the meadow. He says for example:

> Terrorism is overrated.
> Chronic stress is underrated.
> The collapse of Lehman Brothers is overrated.
> Fiscal irresponsibility is underrated.
> Astronauts are overrated.
> Nurses are underrated.

> Britney Spears is overrated.
> Air plane crashes are overrated.
> Resistance to anti-biotics is underrated ... (94)

This phenomenon is apparent every single day. For example, on the last day of 2014 – and then for the whole New Year period – CNN was obsessed with the news of Air Asia Flight QZ 8501's disappearance: unusually so, because the plane was carrying no American citizens. News bulletins repeatedly focussed on what they labelled the 'tragedy' and – in unashamed voyeurism – the passengers.

Why focus so much on this event? Why focus on the passengers? Why not choose other stories? Why not headline instead:

> Still no charges pressed over 9/11: Bush a free man.
> US Government continues to fund terrorist organisations.
> Obama bombs 7 nations in 6 years: Fails to return Peace Prize.

How many children died needlessly on the last day of 2014? How many bombs were dropped for commercial interests? How many lies were told? How much good was done? Not only did CNN not tell us, they made the questions invisible.

News is presented as something essential to know, yet almost all of it is irrelevant to our daily lives. Dobelli challenges us: out of the thousands of news stories you've read or watched in the last 12 months, name one that enabled you to make a better decision about a serious matter affecting your life.

Because news is delivered in separate packets it has no real explanatory power. As Dobelli observes:

> News items are little bubbles popping on the surface of a deeper world ... It's not news facts that are important, but the threads that connect them. What we really want is to understand the underlying processes, how things happen. (94)

Instead we're told about the bad goblin for a couple of days, then he is heard of no more.

It's loosely implied – by the tone of a newsreader's voice, by the motion of an eyebrow, by an occasionally deliberate conjunction of one news story with another – that the news has reasons, but there is never any sustained attempt to help us understand and help us make up our own minds about what these reasons might be.

In High School, Dobelli's history text book specified seven reasons (not six, not eight) why the French Revolution erupted. Yours probably did too. I can't even remember what mine said, it was utterly irrelevant to my teenage life, and my incompetent teachers failed totally to convince me otherwise. As he says:

> The fact is, we don't know why the French Revolution broke out … And we don't know why the stock market moves as it moves. Too many factors go into such shifts … Any journalist who quotes, "… the market moved because of X" or "… the company went bankrupt because of Y" is an idiot. (94)

There are no single causes for anything. There are no single reasons for anything. The world does not exist in packets – yet almost all our officially sanctioned experiences indoctrinate us to believe the opposite.

The news – even so-called quality journalism – continually labels people crudely, without any coherent justification or depth. Celebrity, paedophile, prisoner, insurgent, criminal, mother of three, activist … News-media could just report 'the facts' – and bizarrely often claim to be doing so – but the temptation to embellish – and therefore to pervert – almost always gets the better of them. A tsunami or an earthquake is never just a tsunami or an earthquake – it's always a 'disaster' or a 'tragedy' or a 'mystery'. A plane crash is never just an unexplained event – it's a crisis for the airline, a devastation for the families of 'loved ones'; unstoppable 'tears flow' for the missing passengers …

Neil Postman – a prominent American social critic and author at the end of the twentieth century – makes similar points to Dobelli, though Postman's concerns ranged well beyond news-media to television in general and – by extension – the internet, cell phones and other modern communications technologies. In his most widely-read book, *Amusing Ourselves to Death* (95), Postman argues that TV is turning all public life (education, religion, politics, journalism) into entertainment and is, therefore, undermining other forms of communication, particularly the written word. He predicted – *Amusing*

Ourselves to Death was first published in 1985 – that our 'bottomless appetite' for TV will make so much content available that we will be overwhelmed by 'information glut' – until 'what is truly meaningful is lost' and we no longer care what we've lost so long as we are being amused. He writes:

> Contrary to common belief even among the educated, Huxley and Orwell did not prophesy the same thing. Orwell warns that we will be overcome by externally imposed oppression. But in Huxley's vision, no Big Brother is required to deprive people of their autonomy, maturity and history. As he saw it people will come to love their oppression, to adore the technologies that undo their capacities to think … What Orwell feared were those who would ban books. What Huxley feared was that there would be no reason to ban a book, for there would be no-one who wanted to read one. Orwell feared those who would deprive us of information. Huxley feared those who would give us so much that we would be reduced to passivity and egoism. Orwell feared that the truth would be concealed from us. Huxley feared the truth would be drowned in a sea of irrelevance. (95)

Postman could be describing 2017 not 1985. There's so much information to be had so easily these days, creating the seductive delusion that to find the truth all we need do is turn on the computer or other device, google a search term or two, and hey presto – there will be the answer. The truth. The real thing. But the opposite is true. Try to find out what really happened in 9/11 and the problem is not that the information has been deliberately hidden (though undoubtedly those who planned the attack on the twin towers – whoever they were – have gone to extreme lengths to keep their plans, actions and motives secret) rather the problem is that everything is hidden 'in plain sight'. The truth is there to be seen – and we can each draw our own conclusions according to whatever evidence we can identify and interpret – but it's concealed and confused by thousands more alternative truths: facts, half-facts, opinions, real evidence, doctored evidence, misconceptions, hearsay and plain lies. The meadow is full of goblins fighting each other for a brief sliver of our attention, but it quickly gets so much that its far easier just to walk away, leaving them to get on with it.

Postman makes a very interesting observation that the form of the media – the way in which the message is delivered – powerfully shapes its content. He says:

> To take a simple example of what this means, consider the primitive technology of smoke signals. While I do not know exactly what content was once carried in the smoke signals of American Indians, I can safely guess that it did not include "philosophical argument". Puffs of smoke are insufficiently complex to express ideas on the nature of existence … You cannot use smoke to do philosophy. Its form excludes the content. (95)

Postman might just as well have been talking about Twitter or Facebook.

Twitter is almost a metaphor for modern-day fragmentation not only of communication but of thought itself. If you have any more than a handful of people you follow, your Twitter feed continually hurls disconnection at you, at a rate that is simply far too much for anyone to process or pay sustained attention to. You can't use smoke to do philosophy, and nor can you use Twitter.

Almost eerily, Postman traces Twitter-like technologies back to Moorse's nineteenth-century telegraph:

> The telegraph introduced a kind of public conversation whose form had startling characteristics: its language was the language of headlines – sensational, fragmented, impersonal. News took the form of slogans, to be noted with excitement, to be forgotten with dispatch. Its language was also entirely discontinuous. One message had no connection to that which preceded or followed it. Each "headline" stood alone as its own context. The receiver of the news had to provide a meaning if he could. The sender was under no obligation to do so.
>
> Whether we experience the world through the lens of speech or the printed word or the television camera, our media metaphors classify the world for us, sequence it, frame it, enlarge it, reduce it, color it, argue a case for what the world is like. (95)

The devastating consequence of this information abuse was that the world began to make less and less deep sense – leaving us to thrash about for whatever flake of meaning made us most comfortable. In contrast to the sequential, step by step, connected narrative of the printed page – of books and magazines that told coherent stories transmitting intelligent messages – the new communication media swiftly made the world indecipherable.

The packet trap has rapidly obscured almost everything that really matters. But whether we can see it or not, there is always a process that surrounds any decision – whether it's to buy an egg or to be compassionate. No decision is an island. Nothing in this world is an island. Even islands are not islands – they are all joined to everything else. They just look like they are separate.

I think contemporary news-media are failing in their duty to inform and challenge us intelligently. They are failing to help us see the connectedness of the world. This is obviously true of malicious comics like *The Sun* and the *Daily Mail* (in the UK) but it's also true of every other type of news-media. It's understandable – there is just so much babble these days – and it's not always intentional. But while everything is treated as transient (like Dobelli's bubbles popping onto the surface, out of a deeper world) we are just not given sufficient time to pause and reflect on the meadow.

Journalists state what they think is obvious, basically, whereas they should report events as factually as possible and should then also take the trouble to help us understand the persisting issues that underlie those facts. Instead, at the moment, it is as if even the best journalists want to direct us to agree with their interpretation of the cause or causes of things, rather than lay out the complexities and suggest ways we might want to look at them for ourselves.

Very often journalists want to tell us they have identified 'the cause' of something, when it just isn't possible to do this. For example, what was the fundamental cause of the shootings of journalists at Charlie Hebdo, the French satirical magazine? What could the root cause of such shootings possibly be? Terrorism? Religion? Insanity? The availability of machine guns? Inadequate police protection? Inadequate surveillance of suspected 'terrorists'? Offensive cartoons? The history of Western interference in Islamic states? Politics? Group think? Indoctrination of everyone? Inadequate education? Inadequate attempts to reconcile Western expansionism with Muslim traditions? Inflammatory journalism? Poverty? Alienation and hopelessness in young Muslims who see no future? All of these, and more, might be defined as the 'core problem'. Yet to identify a core is not only arbitrary, it diverts attention from the complexities of life, and therefore from sustainable solutions.

There are always deeper stories and unseen connections, and it is in learning and thinking about these that we can grow as individuals and as a society.

Individuality

An academic colleague of mine, Tamara Kudaibergenov, who lives and works in Kyrgyzstan, recently published a short but highly insightful paper (96). Tamara's paper makes a single point: when assessing potential research studies from Kyrgyzstan for ethical approval, Western-based ethics committees are unethical.

There is of course a range of ways in which ethics committees might be considered unethical, including the usual human fallibilities of power, control and tunnel vision. But Tamara's idea is much more interesting than this. For Tamara, much of the problem is the way Westerners see people as separate individuals.

It's the packet trap once again. In the West we tend to see each other as unique entities: private, independent, islands of humanity, apart from each other. In a way, you can see the Western view as rather desperate. We're born alone, experience life exclusively from our own point of view, we fight our corner against a world composed almost entirely of strangers, and sooner or later we die alone. Life's a perpetually grim personal struggle which sooner or later each of us is bound to lose.

So powerful is this Western assumption that 'the individual' is everywhere enshrined in our culture, particularly in law where our individual rights and responsibilities are relentlessly defined and protected. And if we break the rules it is always we, as individuals, who pay the price.

Ethics committees are enmeshed in this individualistic culture – above all else they seek to protect individual subjects in experiments and studies, particularly when it comes to ensuring 'informed consent'. It has become sacrosanct in the West that not only must every subject in any research project be safe from any possible harm – however innocuous – but he or she must be fully informed of the nature and purpose of the study and any risks involved, and increasingly must have the right to have his or her data destroyed once the project is over.

This is fair enough – if you take the view that society is a collection of private beings with specific personal interests that are repeatedly threatened by the interests of more powerful groups of people – research institutions, government, big business and so on. Think like this and you are bound to create rules to secure individuals' interests.

But if you don't see the human world primarily as seven billion isolated units then your rules will be different. If, instead, you see the human world primarily as groups – families, friends, tribes, villages and bigger – your rules – your ethics and your laws – will privilege the group interest. The group – not the individual – will be the basic unit. And so it is in Kyrgyzstan.

Tamara's point is that whenever a Western ethics committee insists on informed consent from each individual participant in any application from Kyrgyzstan, they are being culturally incorrect, even insulting. In Kyrgyzstan – as in most non-Western cultures – any big personal decision is not made by single individuals, however hard that may be for Westerners to understand. It's made collectively, by consensus, following discussion. Therefore, it is unethical to non-Western thinking for Ethics Committees to insist on individual consent.

By now this will come as no surprise – we know that labels, packets, biases and the rest are everywhere and inevitable. But Tamara's paper takes us to an even more interesting place, where it is possible for us to reflect on the possibility that Western individualism itself is a huge distortion of human nature.

What do you think?

 STOP & THINK FOURTEEN: ARE YOU AN ISLAND?

John Donne famously wrote:

> No man is an island,
> Entire of itself,
> Every man is a piece of the continent,
> A part of the main.
> If a clod be washed away by the sea,

(Continued)

> *(Continued)*
>
> Europe is the less.
> As well as if a promontory were.
> As well as if a manor of thy friend's
> Or of thine own were:
> Any man's death diminishes me,
> Because I am involved in mankind,
> And therefore never send to know for whom the bell tolls;
> It tolls for thee.
>
> How do you see yourself? A single individual? A part of your family? Part of a broader community? A small part of a massively connected world?
>
> Add your response on the Values Exchange: http://thoughtful.vxcommunity.com/Issue/think-stop-fourteen-are-you-an-island/23062

Progress

Our technological achievements over the past 150 years or so have been truly astonishing. We are all of us living in an age that our ancestors, even in the nineteenth century, would have regarded as nothing less than fabulous science fiction: we put enormous metal machines in the air carrying hundreds of us each trip, capable of travelling from one side of the globe to the other in less than 24 hours; every citizen in the world can potentially know what every other citizen is doing right now, given a radio, a TV, or a computer with internet access; every year we know more and more about the basic make-up of physical reality via physics and its associated techniques for accelerating particles; we have mapped all the genes in our bodies and are steadily but surely learning more and more about what makes us what we are physically and psychologically; we have eradicated some diseases altogether with our vaccines – smallpox and polio for example are consigned to history, as far as we know – and life expectancy for people in the developed world is increasing year on year (apart from some indigenous peoples, other ethnic minorities and people in poverty).

We have undoubtedly made huge technical progress, if progress means building ever more powerful machines, controlling our local environments, and understanding how pieces of the world and pieces of us are put together. But is this progress really? Has this astonishing leap in science and technology moved us forward as a species?

In 1996 Carl Sagan wrote:

> Our technology has become so powerful that – not only consciously, but also inadvertently – we are becoming a danger to ourselves. Science and technology have saved billions of lives, improved the well-being of many more, bound up the planet in a slowly anastomosing (fusing together) unity – and at the same time changed the world so much that many people no longer feel at home in it. We've created a range of new evils: hard to see, hard to understand, problems that cannot readily be cured – certainly not without challenging those already in power. (97)

We move forward and at the same time we move backward. It looks like we're doing well then when you look a little closer it looks like we're not doing well. Perhaps 'progress' is one of the greatest delusions of all.

In 1996 Sagan was concerned about the environmental consequences – including human-made climate change – that may be a consequence of our 'progress'. In the intervening years a whole industry of climate science has developed with many thousands of its members completely convinced that industrialisation – and in particular our use of carbon-based fuels – has already warmed the planet and is pushing us to the brink of environmental calamity. Whether or not these advocates are correct is an open question, and should remain so, because the climate is ultimately beyond our comprehension. And – though they are rarely heard in mainstream media – there are many sceptics who claim the science is too flawed, the incentives to say humans are warming the planet too high, the evidence is too questionable and the variables are simply too complex.

But let's set that to one side and assume the climate scientists are right, just for the sake of argument, to illustrate the difficulty in assessing whether or not we are 'progressing'. On the one hand we have the huge machines in the sky, the convenience of reliable private vehicles (which might also be described as 'dependence on') and on the other hand we have so damaged the planet such that – if the most pessimistic climate scientists to be believed – it is already too late to avert catastrophe on a grand scale: massive rises in sea level, devastating changes in the atmosphere that will make us sick and destroy our crops, and greatly increased extreme weather events.

So, have we made progress? Three possible answers are yes, partly, and no. We might, of course, say we have made progress in some aspects of our endeavours but not in others – or that our progress is reduced by its consequences, or that we have not made progress since we have created so much new risk. Yet these answers miss the point about the delusion of progress.

When you are deluded, to ask questions of degree within the delusion is actually to fuel the delusion. The question is: is it really meaningful to talk of progress at all, or is this an avoidable distortion of reality?

Examples help us consider this question: military technology is making progress as it builds increasingly accurate and destructive weapons. But is making more reliable and powerful agents of violence a sensible measure of humanity's progress? Better medicine and better medical technologies are – along with other changes – extending people's lives, but is a longer life progress just because it is longer?

Has nursing made progress? When I first started working in the health field, as a researcher, nurses were campaigning to become accepted as academics, on a par with medics. The campaign gathered steam over the years and it eventually became the rule that to be a nurse you had to have a degree – and to be regarded as a true scholar you had to have a higher degree. But as nursing has progressed to become a highly qualified profession, what has been forfeited? There are many who would argue that a negative consequence of academia's focus on science and measurement is the loss, or at least the downgrading, of nursing as a kindly, caring art. Personal contact and connection with patients has become harder and harder to achieve as nursing has to demonstrate an ever increasing set of professional standards – clinical pathways, care algorithms and rigorous reporting of routine clinical functions. Most patients want their nurses to spend time with them, to care genuinely about them and to try to understand their suffering – yet the emphasis on qualifications, supervising assistants and making sure that all the necessary boxes have been checked has become an impediment to this. Has nursing progressed, or not?

Obviously it depends how you look at it. Progress is in the eye of the beholder. Take any example. As Schopenhauer and Buddhism point out – all apparent progress comes at a price: you build a new house but become stressed as your budget blows out; you work intensely hard on your thesis and you reach your goal, only to feel curiously deflated and anti-climactic as you realise that one of your life's driving purposes is over; you are elated to win the European Cup and yet in a few short weeks you have to start all over again to try to keep it.

Whatever you do there is an 'opportunity cost': just like 'risk management', making progress in one aspect of life means you cannot make progress in another aspect of life you might have chosen instead.

We take for granted that devices like washing machines, vacuum cleaners, mobile phones and computers make our lives better – don't look closely and they are obvious examples of human progress. But stand back, peel off the label 'progress' and what can we see? Vacuum cleaners save time, perhaps, but their presence means we're more likely to end up spending more time cleaning the carpets than we need. Mobile phones allow us to be contacted by anyone and everyone, but the price we pay is less privacy, less free time and less time spent looking up and out rather than tapping buttons to connect with people and ideas we already know.

Another way to see this is to ask: to what problem was X an answer? To what problem was text messaging an answer? To what problem was television an answer? And: what new problems has the invention of X created? What new problems has the computer created? What new problems has modern agriculture created?

Kirkpatrick Sale – author of *Rebels Against the Future* (1995) – is unequivocal:

> 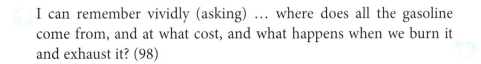 I can remember vividly (asking) … where does all the gasoline come from, and at what cost, and what happens when we burn it and exhaust it? (98)

Sale goes on to point out the uncomfortable truth that so many of us dismiss to the back of our minds, that of the seven billion or so people living in the world at least a billion live in abject poverty while 'less than a billion people … even come close to struggling for lives of comfort, with jobs and salaries of some regularity.'

Sale asks us to suppose an objective observer were to measure human progress, and to ask him or her to judge whether the marriage of science and capitalism has been better or worse for the human species on the whole, and in particular to judge if it has brought more happiness, justice, equality and efficiency. Sale suggests that while the objective observer must conclude the record is mixed, he or she could equally not fail to conclude that '… no social indices in any advanced society suggest that people are more content than they were a generation ago … (there is more) … mental illness, drugs, crime, divorce and depression.'

Whether or not we have made progress is a matter of personal judgement – it depends what frame of reference you choose to bring to bear on whatever evidence you choose to select. It depends how you look at stuff. In the end 'progress' is nothing more than yet another label we pin to projects we like and choose not to pin to projects we don't like. And of course we constantly brainwash ourselves:

> I must do better', 'I must make more money', 'This year will be different', 'Onward and upwards', 'There's no looking back.

The epithet 'there's no looking back' is particularly poignant and often damaging. Because we're designed to try to make sense of things, and because we generally see progress as 'moving forward', we are easily trapped into undervaluing the past.

How is a Fiat Punto progress, compared to a fabulous 50s Cadillac?

If religion can make progress, how is one god better than many? Aren't many more fun?

We are all familiar with seeing things differently as children rather than adults – why do we assume that the adult perception of the world is superior to the child's? How is becoming an adult a progression from being a beautiful, curious, immortal child?

Progressing from 2017 to 1989

It's even arbitrary to judge 'progress' as 'moving forward' – we might just as easily reverse the thought:

> Looking at 2017 and 1989, I can see progress in the move toward 1989.

Bear with the idea that it makes sense to think of a person progressing from 2017 to 1989. In fact, if you were alive in 1989, think about what this sort of progress would look like, if you can.

I was alive in 1989 and I am alive as I write this. So, in my mind if not in reality I can journey to 1989 from 2017, and I can see that journey as progress, if I choose to. All I need to do is stand in 1989, aware of the 2017 David Seedhouse, and ask myself two questions: What have I gained? What have I lost? On one conception of progress – if I have gained more than I have lost, then I might claim to have progressed. Of course, I wouldn't really make this claim, not because 'making reverse progress' is a weird concept, I don't think it is, but because it's so obviously artificial to claim to have progressed in general when all you would be doing is identifying a few packets of your life.

In 1989 I had a smaller house, it was worth less money than the one I have now, its garden was less productive, I wasn't earning much money, I was younger, better looking, fiery, inspired, rebellious, determined, I had more cats, more things were possible for me, I could run, I knew less, I was more optimistic and angrier than I am now (well only a little bit), my best friend was alive and I could talk to him, I didn't have my cats, I didn't have my daughters, I had more potential.

Dependent on how I chose to look at these aspects of my life, selected at random, I can call some of them progress and some not: none of them are objectively progress, they are all personal judgements – is a smaller house worse than a bigger one? Is having less money worse than having a heap of retirement savings? Is youth better than middle age?

'Progress' only makes sense in a very limited way. I have saved for my retirement – assuming I survive long enough to retire – so there is sense in saying that my savings have progressed – but this is only one aspect out of literally countless aspects of my life that I could choose to consider progress or not (I could equally see my savings as indicative of my decline into flaky old age).

By reflecting on 'progress' in this way, we undertake a constructive activity, not dissimilar to Buddhist exercises that ask us to examine our sufferings and those of other people. By removing the labels 'suffering is bad', 'suffering is to be avoided', 'it is better that other people suffer rather than me', 'progress must be understood as moving forward', 'progress is necessary', 'progress is an objective concept', we free ourselves to see new possibilities.

In delusion we tend to see inherited possibilities – conventional goals, pathways defined by others, handed down options – but abandon these legacies and you can ask new questions. How has my suffering helped me grow? How has my pain helped me better appreciate freedom from pain? What has progress cost me? What have I lost as I 'progressed'?

It's exciting to consider the possibility of 'progressing' from 2017 to 1989 because it helps me see the frustrations I felt then as opportunities, as gifts that prompted me to move beyond them. Now I can look at my progress from 2017 to 1989 and think: what's good about this? And then – since I live in the 'present moment' – I can take lessons from my reverse progress. What have I lost that I can restore? What do I have now that I can abandon?

I don't think it's nonsense to say:

> You know what, this 1989 me is in many ways better than the 2017 one. I forgot that, but I can see that in some ways the 1989 David has made progress.

And – weird as it may seem – this should stop us in our tracks and make us see 'progress' in a very different light.

Unless we keep an open mind, 'progress' is a damaging label. If you always have to progress it means you're never perfectly content with what you have. A superficial view of 'progress' undermines now. 'Progress' as a label is a goblin.

Plants

It may seem, in a book directed primarily toward health workers, a little bizarre to include a section about plants. But why not? After all, convention is just another label and plants not only illustrate key themes in this book, but if we look at them free from our typical assumptions, plants can teach us to see the world differently. And seeing differently – seeing more thoughtfully – is what this book is all about.

First of all, as YN Harari (99) and others have pointed out, while we complacently assume that it is we who control plants, there is an alternative perspective. Maybe we didn't domesticate wheat, maybe wheat domesticated us.

Before we farmed the land human beings were hunter gatherers. Like other omnivorous animals, we ate plants (often because the plants wanted us to, attracting us with sweet colourful berries so we would eat their seeds then spread them as they passed through our bodies) and we hunted other animals. We were not tied to any particular place and had no land to tend. So long as food was available to us we were remarkably free: we didn't need money, we didn't need to save, we didn't need to build technology other than weapons, we didn't have rush hours and we didn't need to live the unnatural lives most people in the West live now.

Then wheat got lucky – or smart – take your pick. Out of the hundreds of species of grass that existed, somehow wheat persuaded us to adopt it. We learnt to convert its grains into foods we could eat and enjoy, and so escape (or was it?) a life of eating berries and nuts and wild animals by planting, farming and harvesting wheat grains. We no longer had to (or were able to?) roam to find our nourishment. We could stay in one place, grow wheat, capture animals and farm them rather than hunt them and kill them straight away.

This change was enormously beneficial to wheat. Whether it's benefitted us as well is less clear. But from the wheat's point of view it was the equivalent of winning the National Lottery, week in week out. Wheat no longer had to compete with other grains or any other plants it would presumably label as 'weeds' were wheat to have a human brain – we looked after it, coddled it, protected it from other plants and animals, bred it to make it stronger and more disease resistant – wheat was the teacher's pet and we did everything we could to look after it. We still do.

From the wheat's perspective, wheat domesticated us. We think we're in control of the wheat (and other plants) and yet wheat has tied us to lives where we have to stay in one place to nurture it. It allows us to convert it into products we like – it feeds us – and in return we store its grains, protecting them from the elements, we prepare the ground for it, we distribute its seeds in their billions, we feed and water it and we prevent other species competing with it. Wheat couldn't really hope for a more compliant 'master'.

Most human beings see plants as unintelligent, immobile objects – simple things that just sit there waiting for us, at our disposal, entirely separate from us. Little packets of nutrition or decoration – unaware, unconnected, not really part of any underlying pattern. They fuel the delusion that there is us, and there is nature (as if it really makes any sense to say that we are separate from nature) and we are so superior that it is up to us to control nature.

But, as it is with all our delusions, we have oversimplified reality so much that we are unable to see what's in front of our noses.

I have long cherished a book by Peter Tompkins and Christopher Bird called *The Secret Life of Plants*, first published in 1973. I never tire of dipping into it, for Tompkins and Bird actually like plants, and want to know them for what they are. They write:

> Without green plants we would neither breathe nor eat. On the underside of every leaf a million movable lips are engaged in devouring carbon dioxide and expelling oxygen … of the 375 billion tons of food we consume each year the bulk comes from plants, which synthesise it out of air and soil with the help of sunlight. The remainder comes from animal products, which in turn are derived from plants. (100)

Like just about everything else around us, plants are much more than how they appear to us.

> At the beginning of the twentieth century a gifted Viennese biologist with the Gallic name of Raoul France put forth the idea … that plants move their bodies as freely, and gracefully, as the most skilled animal or human, and that the only reason we don't appreciate the fact is that plants do so at a much slower pace than humans…
>
> The roots of plants burrow inquiringly into the earth … the leaves and blossoms bend and shiver with change, the tendrils circle questioningly and reach out with ghostly arms to feel their surroundings. Man thinks plants are motionless and feelingless because he will not take the time to watch them. (100)

As soon as you look at things just a little differently, plants come properly into view – not as dumb collections of inert cells, rooted to the spot, waiting to garnish a burger, but as intelligent beings in constant motion. Tompkins and Bird remind us that a climbing plant that needs a prop will creep towards the nearest support. Move the prop to a different place and within a few hours the plant will change direction and move toward it. The pair argue that plants must have intention, deliberately seeking out whatever they want, be it sunlight, moisture, food or support. How else can you explain their behaviour? Plants even move towards supports when supports are hidden behind obstacles. It's almost as if they can 'see' through materials we can't.

Plants not only seem to have intent, but they are staggeringly resourceful. Alpine flowers, for example, are so sure spring is coming, even though they lie buried under snow, they develop their own heat to melt it.

The Secret Life of Plants reports research which shows – or seems to show – that plants are acutely aware of their surroundings (why should they not be?) They relate the story of Cleve Backster who was, in 1966, America's foremost lie detector examiner. On impulse, Backster attached the electrodes from his machine to the leaf of his house plant, a dracaena or dragon-tree, to see if the leaf would be affected by water poured on its roots. To his amazement the plant showed a saw-toothed tracing on the machine's gauge, similar to a human experiencing emotional stimulus. He then wondered what would happen if he burnt the leaf:

> The very instant he got the picture of flame in his mind, and before he could move for a match, there was a dramatic change in the tracing pattern on the graph in the form of a prolonged upward sweep of the recording pen. Backster had not moved … Could the plant have been reading his mind? (100)

Backster carried on his research, though his conclusions continued to seem bizarre. He found that there seemed to be an affinity between a plant and its keeper, not dissimilar to the affinity often found between pet animals and their owners (if that is a right word). Backster discovered experimental evidence that his plants showed a positive response when he decided – 15 miles remotely from them – to come home. Similar observations have been made with dogs (101), as most caring dog owners will find easy to believe. My own – non-experimental – observations with my plants in my own gardens are consistent with Backster's. I once went on holiday and left my mature tomatoes outdoors in the hands of an insensitive man who didn't like people, never mind plants. I told him how to water them, 'the roots not the leaves Bill …'. Predictably, he didn't do a very good job and when I returned they were obviously sad, wilting and in parched soil. I felt sad for them too, but had a toddler at the time and needed to unpack, so I reluctantly left them for 30 minutes or so. Remarkably, when I eventually went to water them they had perked up considerably, even though still dry. They were no longer wilted. Egotistically, I concluded that they were simply pleased to see me, and trusted that a drink would not be long in coming. I still cannot think of a better explanation and I have witnessed the same phenomenon on numerous occasions, now I am aware of what to look for.

Essentially, Tompkins and Bird's thesis is that if we fail to respect plants by not seeing them for what they are, then we not only delude ourselves but damage the plants, the environment and ourselves all at once. They point to a phenomenon rife in the twentieth century, when farmers exploited plants and land in the search for cheap profits. They discuss the flat plains of Deaf Smith County in the USA which had for millennia produced rich herbage and soil in balance with animal droppings and dying vegetation. Then – 50 years previous to their book – human farming began: furrows were ploughed, wheat was sown as far as the eye could see and farmed cattle replaced wild buffalo. Progress was taken as read.

In a generation, things began to go wrong. The soil grew less without the natural cycles of plant and animal life and death, so the farmers added artificial fertilisers, but the chemicals burned up the organic material in the soil, upsetting the natural mineral balance. The soil began to dissipate and clog, and erosion produced 'gullies so deep you could hide a tractor in them'. Then, at last, for some, delusion began to dissipate. One farmer, Frank Ford, turned to more natural methods: animal manures, no pesticides or herbicides or chemically treated seeds and his land began to return to health. Ford concluded, 'if you fight nature in farming, you're bound to lose (100).'

Dr Ehrenfried Pfeiffer (100) – an expert on compost – also found through experiment how plants such as beans and cucumbers grow better together while it is sensible to keep beans and fennel apart. Plants behave like this because they are not objects but living beings with sensitivities we do not – and almost certainly cannot – understand. But we should try. As Pfeiffer commented, it is only from our self-centred human point of view that a plant can be labelled a 'weed'. If instead we see them as functional, deeply connected parts of nature, we can learn a lot from them – but we have to see them in context not in isolation: gardeners in suburbia see dandelions as enemies and either dig them up or blast them with weedkiller, yet dandelions help the soil retain its fertility by transporting minerals up from deeper layers of the soil. And it is – or used to be – a common practice amongst onion growers not to weed out leafy plants since they take nitrogen from the soil which can impede the bulbing up of the onion plants.

Much of what was considered shocking in *The Secret Life of Plants* has become mainstream knowledge in the twenty-first century, and organic farming is slowly becoming both better understood and more popular – showing that if you can see past immediate appearance, a deeper reality is slowly revealed (102).

Plants are literally part of the meadow.

Escaping the Packet Trap

It is possible to transcend the packet trap. There's a very simple technique you can use if you want to exercise and strengthen thoughtful reflection. Whenever you feel too comfortable, just ask what is the purpose of this? What's the point of this label – what purposes does it claim and what purposes does it hide?

The next chapter asks this question about health care. If you like you can use it as a template for investigating the purpose of anything.

SUMMARY OF CHAPTER 4: HOW DOES THIS ODYSSEY RELATE TO HEALTH CARE?

It may at first pass seem a little difficult to see how apparently miscellaneous subjects – risk, luck, school, disability, rights, the news, individuality, progress and plants – relate to heath care. But they do, in two different ways.

Firstly, each topic – like almost all topics sooner or later – has direct relevance to health care. And secondly, thinking about each with a thoughtful, critical mind, exemplifies the approach and attitude that all health carers should continually aim for.

The discussion about risk is obviously important directly, since risk has come to dominate the health care landscape, in ways that often run counter to the most humane care (103). Luck is a frequently brought up by patients: 'Why me?' 'It's about time I had more luck' and so on – and this is an opportunity to open up many avenues of discussion about life and its meaning. School – and the

(Continued)

(Continued)

power and control wielded over pupils by teachers and the other 'authorities' – can serve as a continual reminder of the disparities between the health carer and the recipient of care (104). Disability is a powerful label, which has mostly negative effects in health care, and is probably best to be avoided. Rights to this or that are continually claimed, so it is most instructive to remember that 'claims' is all they are – claimed rights are not imperatives, unless they are legal rights – and even these are open to challenge when the case is strong enough. Habitually thinking about bias and selective editing in the news is ideal practice for reflecting on bias in daily life. Understanding that seeing the social world as a collection of isolated individuals is just one way to view it, and is not necessarily how patients and their families see it, is a constant reminder of the importance of recognising how different people's realities can be. Any claim to 'progress' requires explanation and justification – progress does not just happen with the passing of time. And plants teach us that what may seem obvious, mundane and mechanical is – seen with an open, curious mind – mysterious, wonderful and full of hidden depth.

Overall, if you are going to continue to be a thoughtful health carer, then critical thinking and the persistent exploration of life's complexity, is a habit you must develop both in and beyond your working life. Recognising that so much of human life is uncertain, incomplete, prejudiced and selective does make living more of a challenge – it can be easier to accept what others tell us is true, and to conform with whatever social structures and beliefs we just happen to have been thrust into, but if we do that then we turn our backs on our thinking abilities and independence, and we deny our ethical awareness.

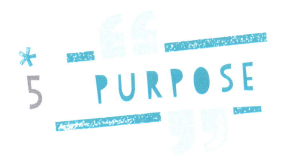

5 PURPOSE

A common factor runs through all the examples we have encountered so far: none of them are underpinned by a clear and agreed theory of purpose.

This may not seem much of a problem. Schools, news-media, risk management, ethics committees and the rest operate routinely, even if they have not worked out their purposes perfectly. And some would argue that values statements and missions adequately define these systems' purposes anyway.

But to me this is a classic example of the packet trap. The point of creating a well thought out theory of purpose is to guide and inform everything you do, within a particular system. A developed theory about 'why we are in business' enables everyone in the system to assess specific policies and actions against the theory, and it also means everyone can check out how everything contributes coherently to the overall purpose.

A theory of purpose is much more than a 'statement of values'. It's a proper account of what should and should not be done, applied to many examples. It's not a code or a list of check boxes, it's a rationale – a justification of practice that cannot be followed by rote, but rather must be applied thoughtfully and intelligently by the people who work in the system (2).

A proper theory of purpose helps everyone see the meadow. Without a theory, fragmentation is inevitable.

If you look only at a portion of the meadow, then you have no need or opportunity to ask: 'how does what I'm doing fit with everything else others are doing?' and 'How does my work fit with and enhance the whole meadow?'

If you don't see the meadow you have no need to ask: 'does the aim of values-based recruitment fit with what we know from philosophy and psychology?', 'Does it fit with the available evidence?', 'What is the available evidence, anyway?' Instead you will blindly chase one small goblin, unsure why or how this might matter in relation to your fully worked out goals. (As we've seen in Chapter 1 – this is precisely what's happening at the moment.)

If you focus only on a single goblin you will have no need to consider 'does my trying to reduce this particular risk create more risks elsewhere in the system?' Or to reflect on whether what you do as a school teacher each day is consistent with a fully-fledged philosophy of child education. Or to ask whether your role in the news-media is to report isolated events, as a set of transient facts offered as daily entertainment, or if it is something more significant.

And so it is with the NHS, and all other Western health systems. There are so many goblins to worry about that the bigger picture has vanished.

What's the Point of the NHS?

The most pernicious problem with the NHS is, most definitely, that it does not have a theory of purpose. This may seem a strange thing to say, given all the codes and declarations which decorate its walls, but it's true. Believe it or not, the NHS is called a 'health service', but nowhere in its Constitution does it explain what the NHS means by 'health'. It's merely assumed that it's obvious.

Because the NHS constantly does what it does, it's taken as read that this is what it ought to be doing. Because the NHS mainly offers clinical services designed to tackle disease, illness and handicap, delivering these services appears so obviously to be its fundamental purpose that few people ask any deeper questions. It just seems to go without saying that 'here's a disease, it's our job to get rid of it'.

For all sort of reasons – court rulings, patient advocacy, organisational reforms, legislation, ethical issues, reactions to unsafe practice (like the Mid-Staffs scandal) (25) – voluminous rules, codes, instructions and the like have been added across the NHS in an attempt to ensure that 'disease care' is delivered in kind and sensitive ways. But – despite all the good intentions – asking 'how can we deliver disease care AND respect dignity?', 'how can we deliver disease care AND ALSO put patients first?', 'how can we deliver cost-effective disease care PLUS offering communication, compassion, caring and so on?', actually feeds the packet trap.

It's as if the human support and kindnesses are somehow conditional. If circumstances allow, staff may add on the ethical niceties and 'official values', but in the end these are not necessary to deliver an acceptable service. 'Respect', 'dignity', 'equality' – at the coalface, when push comes to shove, concepts like these are dispensable, whereas clinical tasks are essential: the clinical work seems solid, evidence-based and needs to be done, the other stuff appears less solid, a matter of opinion, and can be ignored if necessary.

Within the packet trap, diseases and illnesses are seen as separate entities – specific problems that need to be targeted by specific experts. In a way this makes perfect sense – a tumour or a lesion or an eye infection requires competent detection and knowledgeable action. Hospitals are supposed to deal with disease. However, the consequence of the relentless focus on specific diseases and illnesses is to raise the status of disease care above everything else that might be done to support patients' health.

Different sorts of diseases are dealt with by different departments and different specialists with different skills. The type of knowledge and expertise required is thought to be distinct for each discipline. Specialists in the same disciplines identify most closely with each other, and usually regard their work as more important than other disciplines', not least when it comes to securing scarce resources in competition.

None of these factors is unexpected or unreasonable in itself, but the cumulative effect of this culture of separateness causes the system to over-focus on particular, isolated problems at the expense of the many shared goals common to all health care, and which it is the purpose of a strong theory of health to identify.

The best way to shake off these delusions – probably the only way that will work – is to stop seeing everything as separate. And the best way to encourage this in health care – as I've been saying without noticeable effect for 30 years or more – is to explain health in a way that brings clinical work and human support together in a comprehensive theory: a 'theory of everything' for the NHS, if you like.

Health Work is About Creating Autonomy

As soon as disease ceases to be the central focus of health care, the separateness delusion begins to crumble. Change the focus to empowering people or 'creating autonomy' and all the bits and packets start to meld into one.

In my first book I asked the question: 'what is health?' and followed my logic and intuitions through to a powerful conclusion: health is not a medical condition, it's not the opposite of disease, rather health is any set of circumstances that enable people to have fulfilment (2). If they are fulfilling their realistic biological and chosen potentials to an optimum level (taking into account their age and other fixed circumstances) then they can be said to be in the best of health.

On this view of health work, if a person has a disease – or any other impediment – this does not necessarily mean they are unhealthy. It's quite possible to have a disease – any disease – and yet still to be fulfilling some, possibly all, of your realistic biological and chosen potentials. It's also quite possible to have a disability and still be considered – and to consider yourself – in optimum health.

It is only under the delusion of separateness that diseases, illnesses, injuries and so on are described as necessarily causing ill health. On a joined up view, your diseases and disabilities may be seen as a problem or not – it depends how you look at your life and what you want and are able to do with it.

Logically, disease and illnesses are not problems in themselves – they are problems only if we say they are. When our potatoes get mould we call it blight, but to the mould it's a perfectly healthy environment. If we want potatoes then mould is a problem, and we can choose to call the mould a disease if we want. But if we want to cultivate mould – say to make a medicine, or for any other reason – then the mould is a good thing. From a point of view that wants to cultivate mould, there would only be a problem of disease if the mould would not grow.

If the conditions we call disease and illness are problematic only if they are not what we want – if they are problematic only if they are obstacles or impediments to something we want to achieve (freedom from pain, better movement, being able to work, and so on) then health work immediately becomes more than clinical work. If health work is essentially work against obstacles to desirable human potential, then it can – in fact it must – include so much more than clinical activity, and clinical activity can never be seen as the end in itself.

Anne and Dennis

Thirty years ago – half a lifetime away – I wrote about two characters in *Health: The Foundations for Achievement* (2).

Dennis was a middle-aged bank clerk (they had bank clerks back then). He was extremely bored and boring. All he wanted to do was come home after work and lie on the couch, watching sports (Sky TV was in its infancy). His wife seemed happy to make his dinner and clean up after him, but that was about it. Their relationship was not explained in the book, but the implication was that there was little intimacy, physical or mental.

Dennis did have a medical check-up every six months, paid for by his employer. And he always got a clean bill of health, from a clinical perspective. He was advised to exercise more but otherwise he was deemed physically and mentally healthy.

On the face of it Anne was not only unhealthy, but a tragic case. She was in her thirties and had been a successful, up and coming journalist. Sadly, she was in a car accident that left her permanently paralysed from the waist down – there was no cure possible. Not only that but her husband left her saying she was not the woman he married, and she lost her job (there was no internet in those days and her job required her to be mobile).

Naturally enough, Anne struggled with her lot for months, but she slowly rallied. She moved to a specially modified flat – which she really liked – and she got a lot of support from health and social services as she adapted to her new life. Eventually, she managed to get a journalism post that allowed her to work from home, working for a magazine for disabled people. When we meet her in the book she describes herself as content and fulfilled, despite her devastating injury.

We Intuitively See Health as to do with Opportunity and Creativity – Disease and Illness is Not the Opposite of Health

I was excited about my theory of health. I still am, though back then I was excited in a youthful way, and I toured and spoke and taught people at every opportunity. And I made a discovery.

I never wrote this up or pursued it in a scientific way – I probably should have – however, the results were overwhelming. Asked to decide who was the healthiest person – Dennis or Anne – Anne always won, and this was over thousands of respondents. As far as I can recall, no-one ever said that Dennis was healthiest. It was always Anne. Hardly anyone was willing to define her as unhealthy.

And yet, as I pointed out in order to prompt discussion, Anne was a paraplegic, dependent on external support, unable to walk or feel anything below the waist. Anne needed health and social care, I said, so surely she must be unhealthy?

No. No-one would accept that and I am sure this would be just the same today. Anne is healthy because she is fulfilling her realistic biological and chosen potentials, Dennis is not healthy because he is not. Health is not essentially to do with clinical conditions – it's to do with how much movement in life we have. It is to do with whether we are autonomous in the ways we want to be. It is to do with our ability to be creative in life. And this in turn is to do with what I called our 'foundations for achievement'.

To explain this idea, I used to use a simple analogy of a stage, made up by four separate boxes put together as a single block on which to perform, and a fifth box, set to one side. The four main boxes represented 'basic needs', which included 'purpose in life', 'information', 'education' and a 'sense of belonging'. The fifth box – not at the centre of the stage – was for 'special needs', which included nursing, medical and other special support.

To work for health was therefore not just about doing clinical work well – though that is always important – rather it's to identify what assets, for each of the four main boxes, will work best to create autonomy for the person on the stage. In Anne's case her basic needs are covered by her flat and the support she gets – and she quite definitely has purpose in life. She has all the information she needs to live a positive life. She is well-educated, and in fact doing further study. And she has a strong sense of belonging, now she is writing for the disabled community.

Work for health – seen as a connected art – is to take account of as many aspects of a person's life as possible – including understanding her decisions and their sources. Work for health is not therefore only work on bodies and brains – it is work to build the strongest life platforms as possible, and to enable the maximum possible movement in life. Sometimes this does include work against disease, illness and injury – and sometimes this is the most important health factor, if it is the largest impediment to autonomy. But clinical work is never an end in itself. It's always instrumental.

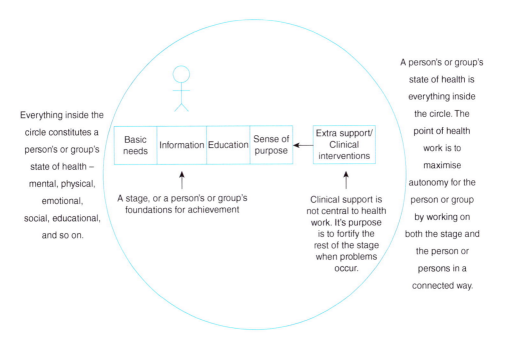

Both the condition of the stage and the person – or group of people – together constitute the state of health of the whole circle. The point of health care is to maximise autonomy by working on the stage and the person or persons. The extra support box represents clinical care – which is sometimes but by no means always the focus of health work.

Figure 5.1   A Simple Representation of Health

Note: more detailed representations of health can be found in *Health: The Foundations for Achievement* (2) and *Health Promotion: Philosophy, Prejudice and Practice* (4)

You have to imagine the fifth 'special support' box being pushed up against the other four boxes. It's not meant to be separate – the reason for the special support is to provide extra help (ideally temporary) not for its own sake but to enable the person to take as much advantage as possible of the other boxes – her life enabling boxes – her foundations for achievement. You provide the special support next to the rest of the stage so the person can jump over to the main stage – and live her life as well as possible on that and the fifth part of the stage, for as long as it is needed.

Seeing health as only the opposite of disease and illness is not logical. Why is disease a more serious impediment to autonomy than ignorance? It's artificial too. Diseases are part of people – part of life. They are never separate problems and they are rarely experienced or tackled without impacting on every other aspect of a person's life, including their families, friends, workmates and so on.

Neither are diseases and illnesses problems *per se*. There are, for example, people labelled as schizophrenic who take comfort from hearing voices, there are deaf people who prefer to be deaf rather than hear, there are people who welcome colds and injuries because it excuses them from work and family responsibilities, and there are people who are happy to have terminal illness.

If you see the world as separate, then it's very easy to focus solely on curing and preventing disease for its own sake, without questioning why this matters. This, after all, is what the health care system instructs its students and practitioners to do: they learn and apply facts and skills to tackle problems of disease and illness. And this is very often seen as the sum of what is required. But the world is not totally separate chunks – diseases are problems not as little packets of reality – they are problems because of what they prevent us doing.

Very few official health systems have ever understood this. Whatever the rhetoric about putting patients first, and all the rest of it, the priorities and the funding follow clinical practice. And this remains a devastating delusion.

There is all the difference in the world between putting this first, to inform your practice:

FIGHT DISEASE AND ILLNESS

And putting this first:

CREATE AUTONOMY

The rhetoric of the NHS is that 'the patient should come first'. However, dependent on which is your primary driver (creating autonomy or fighting disease), 'putting the patient first' will have a different meaning and sustain different behaviours.

FIGHT DISEASE AND ILLNESS

> Don't worry, come what may we will fight your disease – this is what we are trained to do.

Versus:

CREATE AUTONOMY

> We will fight your disease if you want us to, but we're primarily here to support you in many ways, including meeting your basic needs, educating you, giving you as much information as possible even if it contradicts and making sure you feel as connected as possible to what's important to you.

It's hard to overestimate the difference this makes over time. Cumulatively, if all your professional validation comes from your clinical work, this – and possibly nothing else – will colour everything you do, no matter what values statements, missions and declarations are pasted on your workplace walls. If your buzzer goes you will respond since it indicates that something clinical is needed. It doesn't matter what else you are doing – educating, listening, being kind to a patient – clinical need will trump it. This is the culture, after all. It's been subtly and not so subtly instilled over years of training and is continually bolstered in practice: not something that can be changed overnight, that's for sure.

On the other hand, if all your professional validation were to come from your efforts to create autonomy – which in clinical health care most certainly can mean fighting disease and illness – then if your buzzer goes to ask you to help with a clinical need you might decide that if it's creating autonomy, what you are currently doing is more important, even if it's not tackling disease and illness. Admittedly, it's hard to imagine this being the case, but unless the focus of NHS culture changes, then all pleas to be ethical and compassionate and have the right values will remain peripheral.

The difference is that profound. In the end it all boils down to the separateness delusion: **FIGHT DISEASE AND ILLNESS** means that you see a small piece of life as central to everything, at the expense of the meadow. Disease and illness is the goblin. **CREATE AUTONOMY** means you can fight the goblin if that's the best way to enable the people you are caring for, but you won't do so without looking at the meadow first. And once you can see the meadow then, who knows, all sorts of possibilities may present themselves – foundational possibilities, connected possibilities, possibilities that may include disease care but which may also couple it with every other thoughtful way to enable other people.

Here are three examples.

Catherine is the elderly woman we met in Chapter 3. She has symptoms of dementia and now has multiple health issues, one of which is allergic asthma that gives her severe breathing difficulties. Best medical advice is that Catherine should give up her cherished springer spaniel dog, Petra, as there is a risk that it will trigger increasingly severe asthma attacks.

These attacks have already resulted in trips to hospital A&E, and could even prove fatal. However, Catherine reacts very badly to the suggestion, saying that it would be like losing a child.

It is proposed that the health team insist that Petra is re-homed in Catherine's best interest.

 Add your response on the Values Exchange: http://thoughtful.vxcommunity.com/Issue/think-stop-fifteen-catherine/21237

A patient, Rachel, has extensive burns following an accident. She will survive, but there will be extensive scarring and loss of mobility. She is 25 years old, has a PhD and is single.

In your role as a student on placement Rachel confides in you that she is saving up the medicines she is being given so she can take it all at once and commit suicide. She says she trusts you. Only you know.

You have choices. You can work with the situation yourself or you can tell a practitioner in charge of Rachel's intent. Which matters most – trust or safety?

It is proposed that you tell a practitioner in charge of Rachel's intent.

 Add your response on the Values Exchange: http://thoughtful.vxcommunity.com/Issue/think-stop-sixteen-rachel/21235

Farooq is a 48-year-old patient with severe chronic kidney disease and requires haemodialysis three times every week. As part of this procedure, it is required that heparin is administered into the dialysis machine to prevent clotting within the machine. You realise that the heparin is derived from pork intestines. Farooq's profoundly held religious beliefs preclude the consumption of pork. It is very likely that this drug will be present in his blood after the procedure.

> The consultant does not want to risk clotting during the procedure as this could be fatal. Without dialysis for the rest of his life he will die. There are no suitable alternatives. The consultant does not want the patient to be told about this as he is worried that Farooq may refuse treatment.
> **It is proposed that you inform Farooq of the ingredients.**
>
> Add your response on the Values Exchange: http://thoughtful.vxcommunity.com/Issue/think-stop-seventeen-farooq/21236

It seems to me that if you put **FIGHT DISEASE AND ILLNESS** first, then the decision is made for you in each case. In fact, you don't really need to think at all. And surely – ironically – it is precisely this that should give you pause for thought.

It's worth thinking briefly about these three issues. In Catherine's case, there is an assumption that her dog, Petra, is triggering her increasingly severe asthma attacks. Consequently, her health team are insisting that Petra is re-homed in Catherine's 'best interests', even though this is very much not what Catherine wants. The dog may not be responsible for the asthma of course, but for the sake of argument let's accept that she is. If we take the view that **FIGHT DISEASE AND ILLNESS** is the fundamental purpose of health care then we must, I think, try to reduce the attacks and also address Catherine's other 'health issues' and her dementia. Her diseases and illnesses would be the focus and dealing with them would be the priority. But is this intuitive? Does it feel right? Does it really make sense?

If, on the other hand, we choose to consider **CREATE AUTONOMY** as the fundamental purpose of health care, everything changes. First of all, it becomes necessary to balance all the factors in play, since they can now be seen to be obviously connected. Catherine's disease and illness is one part of a complex picture – it's no longer an imperative. What we need to do is consider which interventions (or none intervention) of the many possible will best create more autonomy for her. Of course, it may turn out that she already has as much autonomy as possible, so we cannot create any more for her, in which case we will need to make sure we do not reduce the autonomy she has. Which means, in my opinion, that we should respect her choice to keep her dog, despite the disease risk. This will make her happier. It will make her less anxious. It will treat her with dignity – not as a separate concept but as a natural consequence of working for health in a rounded, holistic way.

Allowing Catherine to keep her dog is not an inevitable conclusion. It might be that her asthma is so dangerous that it's likely to kill her at any time, which will remove all autonomy from her forever. So there is an argument that Petra should be re-homed, in order for Catherine to continue with her life and her other choices, in the interest of her autonomy.

I don't think this is a very good argument, but that's not important. What matters is that placing **CREATE AUTONOMY** as the basic purpose of health care creates richer options, in a more realistic and connected way. Her health carers can choose to focus on her diseases or/and they can look at education, support, different bedding for Petra, new shampoo for Petra, different medications for Catherine, more information, different ways of enabling Catherine to see Petra – lots and lots of options. But if you place **FIGHT DISEASE AND ILLNESS** as the top priority then your option is only to do that, or perhaps to do that with 'ethical add-ons' – for example choosing to **FIGHT DISEASE AND ILLNESS** as the priority while also maintaining Catherine's dignity, though it is not clear to me how you would do that given that disease is your *raison d'être*.

The same applies to Rachel and Farooq. The medical priority for both is first to maintain life, and then to look at further treatment options (in Rachel's case probably psychiatry or psychology, and for Farooq a transplant operation). If you put **FIGHT DISEASE AND ILLNESS** first, then you really have little choice but to think this way – the purpose must be to tackle disease and illness. This, rather than each patient as a whole, is what matters. But place **CREATE AUTONOMY** first and your options instantly expand. You are free to think more deeply about your goals and how to achieve them. There are just so many more ways you can be creative, and so many more ways you can see the connections and influences that make up a real life. It is surely much easier to empathise with people if you see their choices embedded in a life process, rather than be mystified as to why they might choose other priorities over fighting disease and illness. Using **CREATE AUTONOMY** as a first step liberates you as much as it liberates the patient.

You don't have to adopt a vacant list of values either. The first question should not be 'how does this fit with the 6Cs?' or some other pointless refrain, but what do I need to do practically to enable this person to make the best choices for her, in her present circumstances. How can I best work for this unique person's health?

This is not an easy question by any means. Nor are there right answers. Every deliberation will be different from every other, and will depend upon what you bring to it, what the patient brings to it, and what the prevailing circumstances are. There are several techniques you can use to help you (see Chapter 8) – such as tools for systematic ethical reflection when things get very complicated (105) – but in the end it is up to you, as a health carer, to think creatively, deeply, purposively and with as much self-awareness and awareness of others as you can muster.

SUMMARY OF CHAPTER 5

1. The most damaging problem with the NHS is that it does not have a theory of purpose. This may seem a strange thing to say, given all the emphasis on codes, values statements and key words, but while the NHS is called a 'health service', nowhere in its Constitution does it explain what the NHS means by 'health'. It's merely assumed that it's obvious.
2. It is taken for granted that the purpose of the NHS is to prevent or cure disease and illness, but while this is obviously important, diseases and illnesses are not cured for their own sake – they are cured because they are impediments in the way of people living life in the ways they want. A broken leg is not put in plaster just because it's broken, it's fixed in order to free its owner to walk and run.
3. It follows that the central purpose of health care is work to 'create autonomy' – to empower people to live as well as they can.
4. Health is not a medical condition, it's not the opposite of disease, rather health is any set of circumstances that enable people to have fulfilment. If they are fulfilling their realistic biological and chosen potentials to an optimum level (taking into account their age and other fixed circumstances) then they can be said to be in the best of health.
5. If a person has a disease this does not necessarily mean they are unhealthy. It's quite possible to have a disease – any disease – and yet still to be fulfilling your realistic biological and chosen potentials. It's also quite possible to have a disability and still be considered – and to consider yourself – in optimum health.
6. There is all the difference in the world between putting this first, to inform your practice:

    FIGHT DISEASE AND ILLNESS

    And putting this first:

    CREATE AUTONOMY

(Continued)

(Continued)

7. It's hard to overestimate the difference this makes. If all your professional validation comes from your clinical work, this will colour everything you do, no matter what values statements, missions and declarations are pasted on your workplace walls. This will be your priority whatever 'big values' words you are asked to adopt.

    On the other hand, if your professional validation comes from your efforts to create autonomy then you will ask first: 'which is the most empowering intervention I can make?', rather than aim to tackle the disease above all else. The clinical textbook may suggest aggressive chemotherapy for a 73-year-old woman with two primary cancers and local metastases, but this intervention is not necessarily the most autonomy creating.
8. If you choose 'create autonomy' as the basic rationale of health care you will have richer caring options, which you will see in a more realistic and connected light.

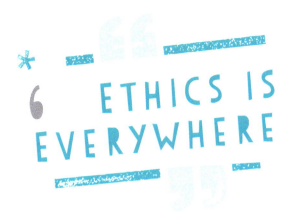

6 ETHICS IS EVERYWHERE

In the last chapter we met Catherine, Rachel and Farooq. For each there was 'an ethical issue': should we take Catherine's dog from her, should we break Rachel's confidence, should we lie to Farooq? The way the issues are presented, with just one proposal per case, makes it seem as if they are occasional dramas – stand out issues that need urgent attention and perhaps special expertise to solve. But this is quite mistaken.

It is widely believed that for most of the time life proceeds in an untroubled stream. To take a general example, most people trust that junior doctors work in a normal, stable environment. Everything's fine. There are no news stories to read. Things are normal. Then, apparently out of the blue, some of them decide to go on strike. The strike – right or wrong, is it ethical? – immediately becomes the focus of intense media and public debate, as if a troublesome goblin has suddenly landed in the meadow.

But this is a delusion – appearance, not reality. Deeper issues are constantly present. When you think about it they must be, or else the ethical drama would have no source. Should junior doctors work such long hours? Should anyone? Are junior doctors being inducted into a damaging system? Does the system wipe out idealism? Is demotivation and cynicism inevitable? What is the purpose of being a junior doctor? Why is ethical reflection and deliberation not a central part of their day? Why are so many disillusioned with the career they have chosen (106, 107). Why is medicine not seen as a creative art? Why is there a culture of bullying in medicine? What should be done about callous mentors?

These ethical issues – and endless more – are constantly present. The only reason they are not seen as such is because no-one is currently labelling them. But that does not mean they are less important than the single goblin everyone's pointing at.

It's astonishingly simple really. We're in the habit of thinking that 'ethical issues' are the 'headline' cases – euthanasia, abortion, life and death choices. So we take a few bits of the world – the obvious bits – and we label these as 'ethical dilemmas' by repeatedly featuring them in books, papers, television programmes, ethics classes and so on. These labels then quickly come to represent all the social realm we consider to be of ethical interest. And – as it always is with labels – they obscure everything else of ethical interest.

In Catherine's case, 'dog or no dog?' may be the question of the moment, but there are many other connected concerns just as difficult to decide. Why do the medical team think they have the authority to remove Catherine's dog? What efforts and techniques have been used to involve Catherine in this decision? What alternative ways are there to manage her asthma, and which would Catherine prefer? What does Petra, the dog, want? Why are human rights and choices more important than those of animals?

Why is Rachel's potential suicide a clinical issue? Is it because she is saving up her medications? Is it because suicide is considered a mark of insanity, even though it is legal and a personal choice? If Rachel were to discharge herself and push her wheelchair under a bus, would that be of clinical concern? What if she just jumped out of the window? (http://thoughtful.vxcommunity.com/Issue/think-stop-six-the-open-window/23057) What are the ethical boundaries of health care?

And for Farooq, why is the anti-coagulant of choice derived from pork intestines? What alternatives are there that do not involve the farming and killing of animals (apparently there are at least two: Argatroban and Fondaparinux – but these are less effective)? Why does the clinician consider medical treatment more important than telling the truth? What deliberation has the clinician done to reach this conclusion? What experience does the clinician have in complex social decision making on behalf of others? How has his medical education equipped him to make this judgement? And if it hasn't, how can this oversight be justified? (108)

It may seem normal to use a medicine derived from a pig's intestine. But it isn't normal – or ethically ok – if you are vegetarian or vegan. Reuben

Proctor and Lars Thomsen, the authors of *Veganissimo A to Z* (109) – an extensive investigation of 2,500 products used in daily life – found that by-products of dead animals are in everything from diet supplements and medicine to sporting goods and electronics. Medicine is one of the most difficult products for vegans to avoid since it is very rare for ingredients to be listed on labels, and most people are simply unaware that the pharmaceutical industry uses dead earthlings so extensively.

The most common animal derivative in the medicine cabinet is lactose from milk, used as a carrier, stabiliser or to add bulk. The use of gelatin (ground up skin and bones of slaughtered cattle and pigs) is widespread as a setting agent in capsules, pills and tablets. And red and pink pills are likely to contain cochineal, or carmine, a dye made from crushed insects.

Very few patients are aware of this. And, according to Proctor, the pharmaceutical industry simply isn't interested:

> They have a totally different paradigm ... They don't have qualms about using animals for testing or in products. (110, 111)

As far as I can discover, using so many animals so routinely in drugs has never made headline news in any paper, magazine or broadcast. It is just about invisible.

No labels. No problem, it seems.

Ethics Education isn't Separate

Early in my career I managed to talk my way into a job as a Lecturer in Medical Ethics, in a large medical school. I was the first ever ethics teacher in a UK university, and at the time quite a few people saw this as a triumph, a small part of the dawn of a more sensitive medical education system. I was hopeful myself, but my optimism didn't last long once I understood the size of the edifice I had been given temporary permission to enter.

I soon learnt that while a handful of the clinical teachers welcomed 'ethics teaching', none of them understood it correctly. At best they saw it as a remedial add-on, expecting me to offer occasional lectures to convince students not to behave 'unethically' (even though I was the ethics lecturer there was no slot for ethics on the timetable). I repeatedly explained that this is not what ethics is, nor would it work, but to no avail.

I eventually created and taught a Master's programme in Health Care Ethics – also the first in Britain – and was able to make a positive difference to a few adult learners, mostly mid-career health professionals dissatisfied with the dominant medical culture. But I found it impossible to make a dent in the undergraduate curriculum.

I was not entirely isolated. There were three or four other 'non-clinical lecturers' (not the best label to have in a hierarchical clinical environment, I have to say). They were also – separately, like me – trying to broaden learning in the School to include sociology, management and computing. Each of us was seen as peripheral if we were lucky, but more often we were simply considered irrelevant.

Whenever I did get an opportunity to offer a 'guest lecture' in a slot owned by one of the heavyweight disciplines, I was almost always introduced as the 'ethics expert'. I got so used to this that I always asked not to be described this way, but the label seemed well-nigh compulsory.

In the end I began my lectures by specifically denying that I or anyone else is an 'ethics expert' – which was one factor for my increasing unpopularity in the Medical School.

> I have no more insight into "being ethical" than anyone else,

I would say,

> And that includes all the philosophers, priests and chaplains who have made a career out of telling us the opposite.
>
> I used to study "ethical theory" but now I have access to the multifaceted problems clinicians have to deal with all the time I realise that this theory is useless. It may be logically quite clever, but since the world you guys are going to work in is not based on logic, all the ethical theory in the world may as well be left to gather dust on the library shelf.

This didn't help very much, since there was such a chasm between what I was saying and what everyone expected me to say. Nevertheless, I persevered for a while, mostly using my Ethical Grid (3, 105) to help students assess complicated, real life problems, using a combination of facts, clinical skill, philosophical concepts (like rights, equality and duty), insights from other disciplines (like psychology, sociology and communication), the understandings of others involved (usually patients and their families), relevant law and as much reason as we could muster. This approach didn't work so well either. The students would complain that they didn't know what specialty I was asking them to study, and most imagined that my job was to tell them the ethical thing to do, so they could make a note of it, for future reference.

The more this went on the more I became opposed to the very idea of teaching ethics as a separate discipline – I even published a paper entitled *Against Medical Ethics* in a journal for medical educators (112), which I have to admit was perhaps not the best career move for a young man on a temporary contract as a medical ethics lecturer.

But I saw it all as so misguided I couldn't keep quiet. I said then, and still think now, that there is really no such thing as ethics (so there can be no discipline devoted to it); that all problems in health care must be addressed from as many different perspectives as possible; that there should be no specialist disciplines at all in medical teaching; and that the only sort of questions clinicians need to ask is: 'is this a problem?'; 'to whom is this a problem?'; 'what would be the best solution?' and 'what do we need to do to make it happen?'

Almost Everything is an Ethical Issue

Many people are intimidated by ethics, thinking of it as something you need a degree in or something for which you need a lot of guidance. You certainly can take higher degrees in ethics, and there is a multitude of scholarly works on the subject – some of which are highly technical. Many academics claim to be 'ethicists' or 'ethics experts' and there are thousands of ethics committees in health care and academia that insist on being consulted before any research or new technique can be approved. From the outside it certainly looks as if there is something special and difficult about making ethical decisions.

But in reality ethical decision making is commonplace. We do it all the time. We're all 'ethics experts' because we make hundreds of decisions that affect others every day.

In my opinion, the best and simplest way to understand ethics is first to recognise that ethics is everywhere, and then use a distinction between 'dramatic ethics', 'persisting ethics' and 'ethics in the general sense'. Of course this is a form of labelling too, though I'm not saying that these three categories are absolute or really exist (one person's drama may well be another's persisting obsession). My labels are merely intended to provide a little insight into how we can, if we want to, knowingly choose to categorise social reality in a helpful, holistic way.

In my lectures and early writing I used to use an image of an iceberg to explain this way of understanding ethics. The iceberg is floating in a sea, with its tip above water and the rest submerged. The tip is labelled 'dramatic ethics' – the only visible part of the iceberg. Underneath, there's a middle section labelled 'persisting ethics' and at the foot of the iceberg there's a segment labelled 'ethics in the general sense'.

You can see the actual iceberg in *Ethics: The Heart of Health Care* (2).

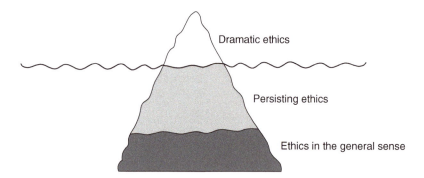

Figure 6.1   The ethics iceberg

Dramatic Ethics

The term 'dramatic ethics' refers to the hard choices that seem to stand self-contained, in isolation from other personal or work issues. For example, if you are caring for Rachel and she has befriended you and shared the information that she is going to kill herself, then you have a dramatic ethical problem. You have to make a decision one way or another. You can't sit on the fence.

Persisting Ethics

However, dramatic ethical dilemmas are nothing more than ethics at the tip of the iceberg.

Because it's much easier – and usually more entertaining – to think of ethics as 'either/or decision making', there is nowhere near enough attention paid to 'persisting ethics' – the issues that permanently underlie the supposedly intermittent ethical dramas. Every one of the diverse topics discussed in Chapter 4 reveals a sea of persisting choices that are just as much ethical issues as those that appear on the surface: wiping out indigenous plants to turn huge swathes of land into fields for wheat; never questioning what 'progress' means; teaching children in schools that success as a teenager ultimately means getting the best grades; thinking of each individual person as an island, while judging broader connections between communities as of secondary interest; treating the news as a form of entertainment, driven by a need for better ratings than competitor news stations; accepting without thinking that natural human rights exist. All of these are of massive ethical concern, yet they are rarely seen or discussed in any mainstream format.

Ethics in the General Sense

The phrase 'ethics in the general sense' refers to deliberation about how best to conduct one's life in general. The person who deliberates in this general sense of ethics realises that all thought and action can and should be the subject of moral reflection. Admittedly it might not be instantly obvious that decisions about whether or not to pass the salt to a fellow diner, or whether or not to continue sitting in an armchair doing nothing, have moral relevance – but they do in this general sense.

To see the point of 'ethics in the general sense' all you need understand is that whatever one does, either to oneself or another person, does not have to be done. Alternative courses of action are almost always possible, and these alternatives can be valued differently and can have different consequences. Dependent upon what you choose to do, you can always enhance or damage your own or someone else's existence, even if only to a small extent. If you are asked to pass the salt at a dinner party you can do this gladly, casually or with obvious irritation – possibly causing the person who made the request to feel more or less at ease. The result of a positive behaviour might be that the recipient will enjoy his meal more, be stimulated into interesting conversation and you will probably have had a beneficial effect on all the diners. Alternatively, if you know something about nutrition and heart disease you might decide to inform your friend of the possible consequence of excessive consumption of salt. You might tell him this nonchalantly, jokingly or seriously – you might even choose to scare him and cause him to feel guilty and anxious about his past habits.

And if you are sitting in an armchair – well, you might be doing something else. In normal circumstances there should, of course, be no compulsion on a person not to sit in an armchair if that is what he chooses. However, the inescapable fact is that other things are possible. By remaining in the armchair (say you just happen to have woken up in it, you don't need to relax anymore and you simply continue to do nothing) you are doing little or nothing to create more of the possibilities open to yourself, nor are you doing anything to enable other people. It's hardly the depth of immorality to remain in an armchair (everyone has to be somewhere, after all) but neither is it the height of morality. You could be doing more. Whether or not to sit in an armchair is a moral issue.

The entire iceberg – or the entire social world if you like – is 'the ethical realm'. And all of us all the time are inescapably within it. Yet the ethics delusion denies it.

The trouble is, if you see ethical issues as occasional and separate, then you end up not considering what is good and bad about the vast majority of stuff – all of it questionable – you define as 'normal'. Every part of our human life illustrates this point, every last bit of it. The sorts of 'ethical issues' highlighted in the news-media are not even the tip of the iceberg – they are merely sparkles of ice on the tip's surface – random choices from millions of other options that might equally be closely examined.

Once you understand that everything is connected, this is blindingly obvious.

My Dad

I have no idea why I think about ethics – or anything else – as I do, but I suspect that – like everyone else – quite a bit of it has to do with what happened to me as a child. I would certainly trace my sense that everything is connected, and that everything is of ethical concern, to this experience.

My father – Charles Donald Seedhouse – was a Biology school teacher. He began to suffer from Multiple Sclerosis in his late twenties, when I was just starting school. He deteriorated relentlessly and by the time I went to the school he taught at, he was in a wheelchair and unable to feed himself without help. Nevertheless, he continued to work.

Whether or not I should have been a pupil at my father's school is very definitely an ethical issue in itself – and sadly it was by no means the only one.

When I was aged between 11 and 14, my father's illness made it impossible for him to continue to work, and he left the school. During the time we were both there, there were numerous distressing matters that could be seen as separate ethical issues, but which it makes much more sense to see as connected like a weave.

For me, one of the most pervasive issues was having to endure personal ridicule for having a 'cripple' as a Dad, and having to suffer hearing some impossibly cruel comments about him: 'your Dad's a spastic', 'your Dad's going to die soon', 'your Dad's a freak', and so on. But even worse, when I was a pupil in the class he taught, I had to cope with seeing him with unstoppably shaking hands in his wheelchair, doing his best to do a good job, but not really being able to, which I was horribly and helplessly aware of. Worse still – and I just couldn't cope with this – he was unable to go to the toilet in the normal way so, from time to time, frequently in fact, in class, he had to push himself to the back of the room in his chair, turn his back to the class, and then fumble to pee in a plastic bottle with a lid, with all my peers in the room.

Terribly for me at my tender age, he was not always able to put the lid on the bottle, with shaking hands, which lead to accidents, sometimes. This amused a lot of my classmates, for reasons I still do not comprehend. And no adult did a thing about it. No-one talked about it and no-one helped in any practical way.

And beyond this there was his increasing isolation from other staff members, some of whom had purported to be his friend. Yet, one by one they dropped away. He couldn't climb the stairs to the staff room and so at lunch and break he just sat in his wheelchair, in his classroom, alone. God knows what the poor man was thinking.

When he eventually left, there was a collection for him and someone decided to buy him a carriage clock and a trolley on wheels. If anyone had really wanted to rub his situation into him, I cannot think of a better way to do it: 'Hey Don, someone can wheel salmon paste sandwiches into your disability room while you watch your remaining, pointless hours tick slowly away. Thanks for your work, Don.'

I saw all this, and felt it constantly, like an open wound, rotting my life. And of course, unlike my peers and his morally crippled colleagues, I understood all the rest of his struggle, which I witnessed constantly: his increasingly spoiled relationship with his wife, his frustrations, his jealousies, his denials, his optimism and his despair, what it took to convert a vehicle to transport him, what it took to straighten his legs sufficiently to sit on the foot rests of his wheelchair (his legs became as stiff as rods, and when I straightened them, several times a day, I know I hurt him, I know I did), what it took to get money to feed the family when he had no job – what it took to cope with a torturous, extended death.

I have no idea how awful it was for him – I can't imagine it – which I think is worst of all.

There are a lot of dramatic ethical issues here. It seems to me, like all ethical dramas, that they cannot be seriously considered without at the same time thinking about the much deeper and broader context within which they sit.

Dramatic ethics: Should the school have continued to employ my father? Should staff have made more effort to see and support him? Should his classroom have had a temporary toilet set up for him? Should I have been taught by someone else? Should I have been counselled? Just a little help to cope with it all? Should just one adult have talked to me about my experience and what I was feeling? No-one ever did.

Persisting ethics: There are so many persisting issues – these occur to me at random as I write. What was the purpose of my schooling? What are all the cruel boys doing now and did Carre's Grammar School make any difference to them? Why does difference – separateness – make it so much harder to be kind? Why did we have no classes on disability in the school? Or about philosophy? Why did so much that didn't ever matter a jot so obsess the teachers there that they ignorantly damaged children by forcing them to do things they did not enjoy and were not good at? Is there really such a distinct difference between 'normal' and 'abnormal' – and who defines it? Why in the West is the nuclear family – in this case my mother, father, brother and sister – considered the fundamental unit rather than the wider community in the school and our neighbourhood? Why – when what is obviously wrong is challenged (as I repeatedly did, one way or another) – are most human beings so very defensive? Why is it so hard for us truly to empathise with others, even when they are next door?

Ethics in the general sense: How should I behave? How should we behave? What is it right to do right now? These should be constant questions.

I wasn't sure what to do about my situation. In truth, I had no idea whatsoever. Maybe I should have asked for help, but I didn't know how. Maybe I should have talked to my Dad about how I was feeling, but I was too shy, had no confidence and lacked the necessary skills. I did have choices but most of my reactions were just that – reactions – rather than considered approaches to an impossibly difficult problem.

As far as I know, the adults involved in this situation failed to address even the most obvious ethical issues, never mind recognise the persisting ones. I assume this was due to a lack of education and insight – and probably they were all too embarrassed and expected someone else to sort it out. But it would have been so much better had they been able to look more deeply at what was happening.

Instead, I was made a scapegoat, which continues to perplex me, even in my late middle age. I was the goblin. The basic problem – for the school – was my behaviour rather than my desperation (I often played truant and was more interested in chasing the prettiest high school girls than eighteenth-century European history). One day – shortly before my father retired – the Headmaster paid a visit to my house. He was annoyed with me. He berated me for my O-Level (now GCSE) grades. I wasn't doing myself justice. I wasn't working hard enough. I wasn't living up to expectations. I was letting the school down. I wouldn't be able to apply to Oxford if I didn't pull my socks up.

He made me feel even worse, even more self-conscious, even more guilty. I think that was his intention. I do wish he had been more able to examine his own ethics rather than castigate mine.

I forgave him, though. There are so many choices, for all of us, that life can be overwhelming. Who has any idea what is really best to do? All we can hope for is that we remain aware of our choices and are able to reflect on them, considerately and creatively, and always in the broadest context.

The Four Principles Fallacy

There is a very popular book about ethics in health care and medicine that exhibits every negative characteristic explained in this present book. The book, *Principles of Biomedical Ethics*, by Beauchamp and Childress, argues that ethics consists of only 'four principles' and tries to instruct the reader in how to apply these (113).

I've lost count of the papers I've read that state – usually with very little argument or elucidation – that 'the four principles of medical/health care/bio ethics are beneficence, non-maleficence, respect for autonomy and justice'. Typically, this is offered as a factual claim: 'there are four principles, you should use them', and that's that.

Beauchamp loosely defines these principals as:

1. Beneficence (the obligation to provide benefits and balance benefits against risks)
2. Non-maleficence (the obligation to avoid the causation of harm)
3. Respect for autonomy (the obligation to respect the decision-making capacities of autonomous persons)
4. Justice (obligations of fairness in the distribution of benefits and risks)

By using them, either singly or in combination, a health carer is supposed to be able to give a satisfactory answer to any moral problem she comes across in her work. Beauchamp admits that she may need 'additional interpretation and specification', and perhaps further rules such as 'don't kill' and 'tell the truth', but essentially the four principles, on their own, are supposed to be enough for all moral deliberation in health care.

Many commentators – including myself – have severely criticised the four-principles approach as a 'mantra of principles', dogma repeated with little reflection or analysis.

The philosophers Gert and Clouser (114), for example, point out that the 'four principles' are little more than checklists or headings and as such cannot produce specific guidelines for moral conduct. There is no theory or justification for the principles, and no explanation about how to use them intelligently. And in the real world the principles always compete in difficult circumstances, yet Beauchamp and Childress offer no advice about how to deal consistently with either theoretical or practical conflict.

Each of the four principles is open to interpretation so wide it's unintelligible to state 'I am following principle X' without further explanation of what you take X to mean. And if you do bother to spell out what you mean more exactly you will find you have gone beyond the principles anyway – thoughtful reflection on moral and practical priorities renders the four principles redundant.

Just think about any real case and try to apply the 'four principles' to solve it.

Let's take Farooq. According to the four principles we have to be beneficent, non-maleficent, just and respect his autonomy. And in order to do this we have to define the benefits and risks (or else we will be unable to balance them), and we have to say what we mean by 'harm' and 'justice'. But we can't do this using the principles. We have to list what we ourselves understand by these things. Not everyone will see it the same way, nor will everyone necessarily see things the same way as Farooq.

But let's give it a go.

> **Benefits**? Dialysis without clotting. Telling the truth.
>
> **Harms**? No dialysis. Possible haemorrhaging. Farooq refusing treatment. Lying to Farooq. Farooq finding out you have lied. Farooq finding out about the pig intestines. Farooq being upset. Farooq dying. Farooq feeling he has betrayed his religion.
>
> **Justice**? Well, that depends on what you think justice is – and the four principles don't tell you.

The thing is, I'm stuck. How do I use the principles to decide what to do? I suppose I could 'respect Farooq's autonomy' (respect what he chooses) but unless I first tell him what is happening he will be in no position to choose, so 'respect autonomy' isn't helpful. Nor does it help me work out if Farooq even wants his personal autonomy respecting, or if he would rather be guided by his family or his church.

The only way I can use the principles is if I first make several decisions without them, which surely makes the whole exercise pointless.

Beauchamp and Childress' four principles are just about the perfect example of the separateness delusion, and the barriers to thinking and perception it creates. It is only possible to believe that three words and a phrase can adequately encompass all there is to moral deliberation if your labels are the size of billboards, plastered all over a huge wall, completely hiding it. You can paste 'justice' to the wall as much as you like but you still have to explain why you chose justice rather than anything else, and you also have to say what sort of justice you are talking about. Do you regard justice firstly as making things more equal or firstly as awarding resources on merit, for instance?

And you always have to remember the wall you've pasted over – for that is where the real complexities are, and that is what you have to see if you are going to offer thoughtful, workable solutions.

{ SUMMARY OF CHAPTER 6 }

1. We tend to think that 'ethical issues' are solely 'headline' cases – euthanasia, abortion, life and death choices. We label these as 'ethical dilemmas' by repeatedly featuring them in books, papers, television, ethics classes and so on.
2. This gives the impression that 'ethical issues' are special problems, separate from everyday life, which is ethically unproblematic. But in fact this is a myth.
3. In reality, every human problem is an ethical issue. Every action we may take that can affect other people has ethical content, and thoughtful health carers should bear this in mind constantly.
4. A helpful way to think of ethics is to imagine an iceberg with three sections: dramatic ethics (the headline cases), persisting ethics (the hidden issues that are the real causes of the dramas) and ethics in the general sense (personal deliberation about how to behave for the best).
5. Any ethical theory that sees ethics as separate from life and human decision making in general is deluded, and should be seen as such by any thoughtful health carer.

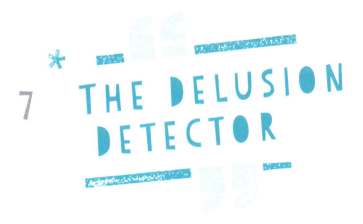

7 THE DELUSION DETECTOR

The final chapter of *Thoughtful Health Care* offers a Toolkit meant to support deeply connected thinking and practice. In order to get the most out of the Toolkit it is important, first of all, to recognise the ways in which you may be deluded.

Types of Delusion

I am hardly the first person to suggest that we are roundly deluded. Advocating curiosity as the best antidote to delusion, Bertrand Russell remarked:

> The man who has no tincture of philosophy goes through life imprisoned in the prejudices derived from common sense, from the habitual beliefs of his age or his nation, and from convictions which have grown up in his mind without the co-operation or consent of his deliberate reason. To such a man the world tends to become definite, finite, obvious; common objects rouse no questions, and unfamiliar possibilities are contemptuously rejected. (69)

Russell's frustration echoes Francis Bacon's memorable list of Idols (115). Once Lord Chancellor of England (in 1618–21), Bacon described four Idols we mistakenly worship: Idols of the Tribe, Cave, Marketplace and Theatre.

Anticipating modern psychology, Bacon calls the first deluding tendency the *Idols of the Tribe*. These are errors of understanding common to the entire human race. Bacon notes that we're rarely content merely to record the evidence before our eyes, rather we need to explain what we see (just as we are driven to label what we see). We prefer some explanation rather than none because we detest it when we can't make sense of things, but as we do so we '… invest … the evidence with innumerable imaginary qualities.'

The *Idols of the Cave* are delusions which arise within the mind of the individual, formed by 'temperament, education, habit, environment, and accident.' Bacon observes that an individual who dedicates his mind to some particular branch of learning tends to become possessed by his own peculiar interest, and interprets all other learning according to 'the colors of his own devotion'. The chemist sees chemistry in all things, and the courtier 'ever present at the rituals of the court' unduly emphasises the significance of kings and princes.

The *Idols of the Marketplace* are errors caused by the constant impact of words used without attention to their meaning – there are tens of examples in Chapter 1. One consequence of the *Idols of the Marketplace* is that we frequently talk at cross purposes without realising it, because we falsely assume that the meaning we give to our words is the same meaning everyone else gives to them.

The *Idols of the Theater* are 'due to sophistry and false learning'. Bacon says these idols are built up in the field of theology, philosophy and science. Because they are defended by learned groups they are accepted without question by the masses. Once these 'false philosophies' have 'attained a wide sphere of dominion in the world of the intellect' they are no longer questioned and – as we've seen throughout this book – our own age is no different from Bacon's.

Guided by Russell and Bacon, I think it is helpful to think of our delusions in three types, and to keep these always in mind:

1) Delusions Created by Our Human Make Up

We are limited in what we can physically experience of reality and – until we invented science and technology – were only able to know the world as it appears to our senses (which are very different from Iggy's, and presumably the goblin's as well). This very understandable delusion is that the world that appears to us is the world that really exists, and that we all see it in exactly the same way. But science, philosophy and psychology – arguably all disciplines – tell us that this is not true.

In all sorts of ways – as experiments in psychology show – what we think we see isn't what is really out there. This is probably the simplest example of all – you can find more in *The Muller-Lyer Illusion (How it Works)* (116):

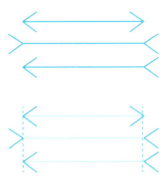

Figure 7.1   The Muller-Lyer illusion

Tom Vanderbilt gives a further, powerful example. He describes a game of American football which took place in 1951. There were a lot of penalties, injuries and rough play.

Shortly after the game, two psychologists interviewed students, showing them film of the game. They wanted to know, 'Which team do you feel started the rough play?' Responses were so biased in favour of the team each set of respondents supported that the researchers concluded:

> The data here indicate there is no such "thing" as a "game" existing "out there" in its own right which people merely "observe".

Everyone was seeing the game they wanted to see. Which to many psychologists would be an instance of 'cognitive dissonance' – where '… people cognize and interpret information to fit what they already believe.' (117)

To Russell, it would be one example of how our unique human experiences – physical, social and emotional – combine with circumstances outside us to create a different reality for each one of us.

2) Delusions Created by the Way We Interpret – or Label – the Reality We Can Experience

This phenomenon is everywhere in human society, and is a central theme in this book. The delusion in this case is that the world as we have labelled it is the world that really exists. There are examples everywhere.

3) Delusions We Create for Others, Deliberately Attempting to Delude

Examples abound, most commonly involving repeated misrepresentation and falsehoods – propaganda designed to make us believe what other people want us to, for example that our own nation is more righteous than other nations. This delusion is like black magic causing us – albeit in a different way from 1) and 2) above – to believe that the world that is presented to us is the world as it really is.

Indicators of Delusion

While we humans are often content to be deluded, if you don't want to be, or if you want to be more aware of possible delusion, there are certain indicators you might like to remember. All of them – one way or another – emanate from the delusion of separateness.

Delusion Indicator 1): There's No Evidence for a Claim – or the Evidence Can Be Interpreted in Multiple Ways and There's No Means of Deciding Between Them

This delusion proliferates in religion, mental illness and the insistence that humans are causing climate change – and in a lot else too. These are big issues, beyond the scope of this book. But we're only interested in noticing 'red flags' at the moment – indicators that tell us we need to be sceptical about what we accept.

In the case of religious belief there's no question. There is no evidence that there is a god, full stop. There is faith – and that's fine if you want to believe – but there is no evidence of anything that cannot be explained in other ways than claiming a deity exists.

In the case of 'mental illness', there is certainly a lot of evidence of mental and emotional distress, indeed this seems to be central to the human condition. But it's not necessary to call this 'mental illness' and label it in all the ways it's currently labelled. There's a whole taxonomy of 'mental illnesses' – officially in the DSM (118) – but this taxonomy is highly disputed, and many practising health carers shun it altogether (15).

And – regardless of the apparently unshakeable consensus of most contemporary scientists – this is equally true of the speculation that humans cause climate change. While the mainstream view is widely accepted, it is by no means wholly accepted and there are many thoughtful analyses of why human-caused climate change is itself a delusion (119). Yes, there is evidence of climate change, but the same evidence can be interpreted in lots of different ways, and there is contradictory evidence too. There is no way finally to prove that the orthodox view is right and the others are wrong: the climate of a planet is just too complicated for that (120).

To view a thoughtful film that challenges the current orthodoxy you might want to take a look at *The Great Global Warming Swindle*, by Martin Durkin. His sensible documentary suggests that scientific opinion on climate change is influenced by funding and political factors, questions whether scientific consensus on global warming exists, and shows – in my opinion beyond reasonable doubt – that CO2 is nothing more than a goblin (121).

In the end it doesn't matter whether you believe the 'human caused climate change believers' or the sceptics. All that matters is that you are aware that there are always many ways to view complex phenomena, and it is always worth exercising caution, and thinking for yourself. I took the trouble to look into the climate change debate over a couple of weeks – and was inundated with data and claims that were very difficult to process coherently (making it potentially tempting simply to accept the consensus – even though I am congenitally inclined to do the opposite). Eventually, I came to the conclusion that the case for human-caused climate change is extremely unlikely to be true – not least because (to my astonishment) it turns out that CO2 (said to be the chief culprit) comprises just 0.054 per cent of the Earth's atmosphere, and human activity contributes less than 1 per cent or 0.0000054 per cent of this amount. Plants, animals and the oceans produce much more CO2 than we do, and the sun and water vapour have a massively greater influence on the earth's temperature than CO2.

I don't know what's true but I do know that people's motivations are highly complex, and so is reality. So I will continue to think for myself, as we all should.

Delusion Indicator 2): You have Beliefs That are Logically Inconsistent but you Believe Them Anyway – you are Using Doublethink

While logic is not a paramount rule of human life – we're inconsistent beings, after all – if you think you can be or do two completely incompatible things at once then this is a very clear indicator that you are deluded.

George Orwell coined the concept of Doublethink in his dystopian novel *1984* to highlight the phenomenon of people simultaneously accepting two mutually contradictory beliefs as true, unaware that there's any conflict (122). Doublethink – it seems to me – is an inevitable outcome of habitually and artificially separating the world into unrelated packets. It makes it so much more likely that illogical beliefs will appear compatible if their true connections are disguised.

Apparently, one of the hardest to see examples of Doublethink is our treatment of non-human animals. Most people like to think of themselves as animal lovers – in the UK for example about half of all households keep pets (123) – and yet it's estimated that only 2 per cent of the UK population is vegetarian (will eat dairy and eggs) and less than 1 per cent is vegan (will not eat or use any animal matter). So it seems that around 63 million British animal lovers are happy to eat them, which is surely more than a little weird.

Here's the Doublethink spelt out:

> I'm kind to animals and I'm interested in their welfare. I keep pets and look after them really well. Sometimes I give money to pet charities. I eat animals that have been farmed and/or killed for me and I eat their products – milk, butter and cheese – they have been forced to give to me against their will.

I'm sure we've all seen people putting money in animal charity collection boxes with one hand, while eating a beef burger with the other. But even staring absurdity in the face, most of us don't notice a problem. We only see it once we're ready to. Until then we flick it away: 'pets are different', 'pigs are meant to be eaten', 'we have to have our protein', 'all farmed animals are treated well', 'you can slaughter animals humanely', and so on.

This is a perfect example of the packet trap in action: there's one wrapped packet for livestock and another for Fluffy and Fido, and these packets are somehow thought to be different in kind. Clearly this is a false belief – pigs, for example, are more intelligent than dogs (124, 125), all animals wish to survive, and feel fear and pain. Other than habit and denial there's no reason not to eat Fido and housetrain Porky – but, in delusion, it doesn't appear that way to us (126).

Here's how it breaks down (apologies for stating the obvious, to those who can see it). First of all, the Doublethink itself: you cannot be kind to animals and interested in their welfare and eat them at the same time, you just can't. If you eat an animal that's been killed for your pleasure not only do you have no regard for its welfare, you have acted contrary to its welfare. Even if the animal has been kept in the most delightful circumstances and been allowed to express all its natural behaviours in an environment that is totally natural for it, you cannot kill it and be kind to it at the same time, just as you cannot shorten a human being's life against its wishes and be kind to it.

In fact, most animals we use are farmed in appallingly cruel conditions and even the most 'organic produce' is killed young (the meat is more tender and you don't have to keep paying to feed it or pay the vet once it's dead). But that is not of present concern. Rather – to avoid delusion – we need continually to hold in mind that it's our labelling and artificial separation of reality that means we can hold contradictory ideas simultaneously – not reality itself.

Jeremy Campbell, in his book *The Impossible Machine* (127), gives an eloquent account of how we often form our stories out of 'flimsy or contradictory data', yet each of us locks onto our story, even 'in the face of devastating logical argument'. It seems that once we have a story, we're not given to re-examining the evidence for it.

Dr Melanie Joy – a psychologist with a career-long interest in our strange Doublethink over animals – calls our animal delusion 'carnism': the belief that animal products are good for us, and that it is ethical to farm and kill animals. She says we pay for our 'carnism' with our 'hearts and minds', as we experience 'dampened empathy and diminished objectivity' (128). Our conditioning to accept that 'the myths of meat and dairy are the facts of meat and dairy' is the perfect fuel for sustained delusion. We come to believe these falsehoods are true because of their ubiquitous institutionalisation – in education, business, religion, government, law, finance and medicine. As she points out, when we're born into a system that looks overwhelmingly normal it is overwhelmingly difficult not to internalise the falsehoods – 'surely so many institutions can't all be wrong?', we mistakenly surmise. This internalisation is so powerful that we don't even have to articulate the thought that eating animals is a good thing, it just seems to be a fact of life.

Joy explains that this stunning delusion is based upon three main elements: justification of the practices using myths, denial because we make sure that the farming and slaughter are invisible and cognitive distortion where we see the exploited creatures as abstractions – 'just another pig' for example, rather than a unique creature with emotion, personality and intention. Put it all together, and carnism blinds us to the absurdities that surround us in every supermarket, a perfect example of which is the well-known brand of cheese called 'Laughing Cow' (129). I'm sure no cow finds it amusing to be made constantly pregnant, to have its male children forcibly removed and killed soon after birth, or to be summarily slaughtered once its milk productivity declines.

I recently wrote to the Happy Egg Company (130). According to their website the welfare of their hens – which they call 'our girls' – is their primary value, 'It's about doing everything we possibly can to make sure they have happier lives …' I asked them what they do with the hens once they stop laying. The Happy Egg Careline replied:

Hi David,

Thank you for your email to us here at the happy egg co.

We put the care of our hens at the forefront of everything we do, which includes how we care for them at the end of their laying life. When our girls no longer produce eggs we can sell to the supermarkets they are taken to our facility where they are exposed to a non-aversive gas to put them to sleep. This all happens in accordance with guidelines laid down by the RSPCA's Freedom Food Scheme and the Humane Slaughter Association.

> We sincerely hope this is enough to assure you that we do all we can to make this process as humane as possible. If you have any further questions please do not hesitate to contact us, we will be more than happy to help.
>
> With kindest regards
>
> the happy egg co.

Our girls? Put to sleep? Humane? Non-aversive gas? I'm pretty sure all sentient oxygen breathing beings have an aversion to being deprived of it, whatever words you use to fool yourself (131).

Our girls go to gas chambers we love them so much. Labels, delusion and separateness.

How do we escape the hold of this deranged and violent ideology? Well, as with all similar violent ideologies, we must make the effort to become aware, and then we must take action. And one of the very first things we should be habitually aware of is that nothing in the social world is neutral. Everything that goes on is informed and shaped in deep and subtle ways, most of which we are unaware of.

Making the causes of our behaviours and beliefs visible is central to our awareness. Paul McCartney, the ex-Beatle musician, is credited with saying, 'if slaughterhouses had glass walls, we would all be vegetarian' (123). This surely would be eye-opening to many. But it's not just the practical effects of our delusion we need to see through, it's the constant presence of the hidden forces, the unseen ideologies, that we desperately need to expose. You didn't just grow up eating meat because it really is normal, natural and necessary, you did it because you were born into a social world where barbaric cruelty is everywhere and normalised as a positive, laudable lifestyle choice.

Joy quotes Voltaire, who said 'if we believe absurdities we shall commit atrocities'. And she talks of the common threads that run though all violent ideologies – domination and subjugation, just because we can. Sadly, examples are everywhere in human history (slavery, racism, discrimination against women, the forced indoctrination of children) and most remain in our present too.

One event that has terrified and mystified me for years, shows not only the depth of humans' cruelty to each other, but the ease with which we embrace truly senseless ideas and actions. The *Kristallnacht* or 'the Night of Broken Glass' was a night in November 1938 where German soldiers and civilians enthusiastically rampaged the streets, smashing the windows of Jewish shops and businesses throughout Germany and the newly acquired territories of Austria and Sudetenland. In an orgy of destruction and hatred, Jews were freely attacked in the street, in their homes and at their places of work and worship. At least 96 Jews were killed and hundreds more injured, more than 1,000 synagogues were burned (possibly as many as 2,000), almost 7,500 Jewish businesses were destroyed, cemeteries and schools were vandalised, and 30,000 Jews were arrested and sent to concentration camps (132).

While this is horrible enough in itself, much worse is the willingness of the German vandals to wreck, maim and kill other German people – people obviously just as human as them. I'm not sure if the psychological patterns are sufficient to explain this. As Dr Melanie Joy says – every violent ideology has the same or similar roots: denial that the perpetrators are doing anything wrong, justification of actions by the use of myth rather than fact (Jews were said to be not fully human, for example), making the actions and the victims invisible if possible (prison camps were kept away from centres of population) and cognitive distortion (Jews are different, it's just a Jew). Surely this is part of the explanation, but I think there must be more.

Perhaps the fundamental basis for Doublethink is that most of us really don't care. Maybe the simple truth is that we're all basically selfish and don't give a damn so long as we're doing alright. So long as we're happy with our myths, so long as we can achieve the petty successes that society tells us we should covet, so long as we can do what everyone else does and believe what everyone else believes, we're safe. It's almost as if most of us are happier when we're deluded, because that way we don't have to think, we don't have to choose for ourselves and we don't need to trouble ourselves or others with awkward questions. We simply pick up a pitchfork, light a flaming torch and race to the meadow with the rest of the mob, snarling and drooling in pursuit of the goblin.

So long as we keep as much of the world as possible in disconnected chunks in our minds, then we can avoid serious thought, and preserve the status quo. And we certainly seem to protect our disconnects with a vengeance in many aspects of our lives. Apparently we love children yet we allow 20,000 plus a day to die of poverty (133). We like to think we are charitable and yet the evidence shows most of us will walk past a stranger in need (134). We talk about equal rights and at the same time allow large companies to evade tax (135). We consider ourselves peace loving and yet we spend trillions of dollars on weapons, and regularly invade other countries using fabricated justifications (136).

The challenge for all of us is to recognise as many 'disconnects' as we can, and help others to do the same.

It's time to start thinking.

Delusion Indicator 3): There's No Coherent Explanation for the Packets of Information you are Receiving

This phenomenon is glaringly noticeable in news-media, Twitter, the internet and the schooling of children – but it's just as true of the information we receive in general. There's far too much of it to process in any deep way, and it's hard to see how to improve things – other than to acknowledge that if we think we truly know what's going on then we are most definitely deluded.

The truth is that most of us are entirely ignorant about almost all of the world around us, yet we act as if we're experts at life and have everything under control.

'The trouble with the world,' Bertrand Russell once quipped, 'is that the stupid are cocksure while the intelligent are full of doubt.' (137)

According to Steven Mazie at Big Think, 'ignoring our ignorance and assuming we know much more than we actually do seems to be a universal human tendency ...' (137).

This is obviously true. As I look around the room I'm working in I am, I admit, completely ignorant about almost all of it, just like everyone else. There are lights on but I have no idea what electricity is nor how it gets into my room. There are windows but I know very little about how their sheets of glass are manufactured. There is a table and ornate chairs, but I haven't a clue how their patterns were made. There are door handles but I don't know what they are made from nor how they operate. There is a radiator which warms the room but I just don't know what is inside the radiator and if it were to go wrong I would be unable to fix it myself. The doorbell, the sash windows, the light switches, the tiles, the coat stand: what are they made of? How do they work? What discoveries in science and technology led up to them? I do not know their stories and I do not know their connections. I am an ignoramus in my own home. How can I realistically expect to have any meaningful grasp of the deluge of information at my fingertips on my computer?

On the BBC homepage at the moment (9.32am GMT, 30 June 2016) there are three headlines:

> Michael Gove to stand for Tory Party leadership
>
> Obama: Brexit will freeze investment opportunities
>
> Motorway hard shoulder plans are dangerous, warn MPs

Obviously, I can click the links to find out more, but I won't find out much more because of the amount of information needed to get a proper sense of what's really going on, and because of the disconnect. Right now I have never even heard of Michael Gove – I know nothing about him other than that he is apparently a Tory member of the UK parliament. I know Brexit refers to a recent referendum in Britain where a narrow majority voted to leave the European Union (about which I also know very little), but I don't know what investment President Obama is referring to, nor do I know why it must freeze.

As for the hard shoulders, I know what a hard shoulder is – a lane on the left of motorways where drivers can stop in emergencies – but I have no idea of their history nor why so much space must be left free on a motorway, and to be honest I'm not very interested. Apparently, the new plan on some busy motorways is to allow drivers to use the hard shoulders permanently, to ease congestion. I feel I should have an opinion on this (do I agree with it or not?) but I don't have sufficient information to decide either way. The BBC article lists some pros and cons, but I am too ignorant to weigh up the costs and benefits (more road space versus less safety – what formula should I use to decide between these? Are there alternative formulae? Is this decision something that can be calculated or is it essentially vague?). I just don't know enough. Any judgement I might make would be out of the blue – a punt about a random issue I'm not qualified to consider – and yet I'm sure most people would be happy to put forward an opinion, and be confident that theirs is the right answer (exactly this happens all the time on the Values Exchange).

Oh, and what is ignorance anyway? It isn't – as you might expect by now – simply a lot of empty buckets waiting to be filled. According to Cornell psychologist David Dunning, ignorance is not simply an absence of knowledge – after all, we can easily discover facts these days – rather it is a lack of insight into the degree and reality of our own ignorance: real ignorance is ignorance of the extent to which we are ignorant.

Dunning's antidote – which we might add to the Toolkit in Chapter 8 – is to:

> … be your own devil's advocate: to think through how your favored conclusions might be misguided; to ask yourself how you might be wrong, or how things might turn out differently from what you expect. It helps to try practicing what the psychologist Charles Lord calls 'considering the opposite.' To do this, I often imagine myself in a future in which I have turned out to be wrong in a decision, and then consider what the likeliest path was that led to my failure. (137)

Self-awareness, which is a vital part of our anti-delusion toolkit, must include a realistic awareness of the impossibly huge amount of everything we don't know, compared to the infinitesimally small amount of the universe we can be reasonably sure of (138).

And we really must stop being so complacent about our favoured beliefs and intuitions. As Dan Ariely says:

> We have very strong intuitions about all kinds of things. Our own ability, how the economy works, how we should pay school teachers. But unless we start testing those intuitions, we're not going to do better. (139)

Questioning assumptions, curiosity, scepticism, looking for deeper patterns and connections – it's probably our best bet against delusion.

Delusion Indicator 4): You're Told to Believe That Only One Conclusion Can Possibly Be True

There is no doubt that we know facts about the world. We know how to build skyscrapers, massive bridges, spaceships, computers and particle accelerators. We know how to engineer genes, transplant body parts successfully, clone living beings and fertilise human eggs outside human bodies. These are amazing achievements which require vast and precise knowledge about the world. If we didn't know what we know we could not enjoy the technologies we do.

But just because we know a lot that does not mean we are right about everything, and we should always be sceptical – especially when we are told that there is only one conclusion about highly complex phenomena. As a matter of fact, most human ideas and beliefs have been shown, in one way or another, to be wrong. Since our understanding is always evolving, and the sum of our knowledge always expanding, nearly all ideas will become wrong, including our current world views (138).

The history of science offers countless examples, including the belief that the Earth is the centre of the universe, that light moves through 'the ether', that life generates spontaneously, that landmasses on Earth are static, that diseases are caused by bad air – known as 'miasma', that alchemy was possible (Isaac Newton was a famous alchemist) and that homosexuality could be cured. These were not crackpot theories, rather they were generally accepted scientific truths, and were studied and taught as such.

Contemporary candidates for scientific truths that will turn out to be wrong include – in my opinion – human-caused climate change, the theory that there are specific genes for specific mental illnesses (140), the belief that there is a 'gay gene' and the Big Bang hypothesis meant to explain the origin of the universe. Maybe I'm wrong, but even if I am it is surely better – and entirely in keeping with the history of science – never finally to accept that there is a single truth about anything (141).

Delusion Indicator 5): You're Told That 'The Evidence Speaks for Itself'

This delusion is similar to number 4, and the same examples apply. But in this case there are theoretical reasons why the evidence cannot speak for itself. Firstly, any piece of evidence must be pulled out of a vast sea of other evidence. So, for example, pointing with certainty to a particular behaviour as firm evidence of a mental illness ignores all other evidence that might have a bearing on the conclusion. Secondly, all evidence has to be interpreted by human beings, according to our particular backgrounds and circumstances. What might appear to be certain evidence of depression to a person from one culture may appear to be a normal state to a person from another culture. For example, in India, a wide range of distress is categorised as 'depressive disorder', whereas in Japan, the very idea of mental illness is unacceptable and few people will admit to having it (142).

Delusion Indicator 6): Value Judgements are Presented as Objective Truths

People asserting that their opinion is a fact happens constantly, all around us. This book is full of examples, and it almost always comes down to labelling. This person is 'unethical', a 'genius', a 'bad influence', an 'anarchist', a 'martyr', a 'prophet', an 'explosive personality' – the list is endless.

It can be very difficult to spot this delusion – well, after all, it is a delusion. However, I find that the best approach, when someone says something they personally value is true for everyone, is to ask 'how would you prove what you say to a Martian who knows nothing about our world?' 'What experiment could you conduct to prove beyond all doubt that this is not your label but a reality that will be seen in the same way by all human beings?'

As Richard Dawkins has written:

> … there's all the difference in the world between a belief one is prepared to defend by quoting evidence and logic, and a belief that is supported by nothing more than tradition, authority or revelation. (143)

Delusion Indicator 7): People are Offering you Simplistic, Separated Reasons as Explanations for Vastly Complex Phenomena – 'The Core Problem', 'The Basic Cause' …

If they tell you your boiler needs a new pump then, if you trust them, believe them. If they tell you that leaving the European Union will increase social cohesion, or that the key to a more thoughtful education system is 'user pays' or that an increased level of CO_2 is the basic cause of global warming, then shake your head, walk away and work it out for yourself.

Delusion Indicator 8): You Think you are in Control of Your Life

We all do. We are all affected by the most extreme delusion of all. We think we can manage reality like balancing a bank account. We think we make our own decisions, uninfluenced. We think we can groom our children to become what we want them to be. We think we're going to live forever.

What do you have control of?

Do you have control of the tides? The weather? The climate? Krakatoa? The exchange rate? Your partner? Other road users? School curricula? The stories you are told? Other people's violence? Your emotions? Your body's immunity to disease and illness? The moon? Your next job? The success of your business? Your parents? The ingredients in the cans of soup you buy from the supermarket? Your desires? Your pain? History? The present? The future? Political decisions? The law? What others think of you? The wind? Your dreams? Your demons?

We will see in the last chapter that we do have some control – we do have some power, but only if we are aware of our propensity for delusion, and only if we are willing to accept our limitations and imperfections.

Put all eight indicators together and you're absolutely guaranteed that there's delusion going on.

It is possible to get past some delusions, even if it's impossible for us ever to be free of them all. The final chapter offers some strategies you might like to try out.

{ SUMMARY OF CHAPTER 7 }

There are eight ways to detect delusion, which all thoughtful health carers should always have in mind.

> DELUSION INDICATOR 1): THERE'S NO EVIDENCE FOR A CLAIM – OR THE EVIDENCE CAN BE INTERPRETED IN MULTIPLE WAYS AND THERE'S NO MEANS OF DECIDING BETWEEN THEM
>
> DELUSION INDICATOR 2): YOU HAVE BELIEFS THAT ARE LOGICALLY INCONSISTENT BUT YOU BELIEVE THEM ANYWAY – YOU ARE USING DOUBLETHINK

DELUSION INDICATOR 3): THERE'S NO COHERENT EXPLANATION FOR THE PACKETS OF INFORMATION YOU ARE RECEIVING

DELUSION INDICATOR 4): YOU'RE TOLD TO BELIEVE THAT ONLY ONE CONCLUSION CAN POSSIBLY BE TRUE

DELUSION INDICATOR 5): YOU'RE TOLD THAT 'THE EVIDENCE SPEAKS FOR ITSELF'

DELUSION INDICATOR 6): VALUE JUDGEMENTS ARE PRESENTED AS OBJECTIVE TRUTHS

DELUSION INDICATOR 7): PEOPLE ARE OFFERING YOU SIMPLISTIC, SEPARATED REASONS AS EXPLANATIONS FOR VASTLY COMPLEX PHENOMENA – 'THE CORE PROBLEM', 'THE BASIC CAUSE' ...

DELUSION INDICATOR 8): YOU THINK YOU ARE IN CONTROL OF YOUR LIFE

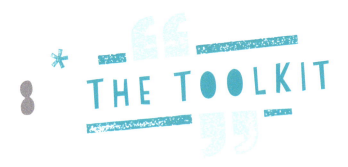

Thoughtful Health Care

This book has been a journey across just a few of the host of ways where we see incompletely.

It's totally understandable that when we're confronted with a problem, we isolate it from other problems. Unless we do this we simply cannot work out how to solve it. Unless we set boundaries to a problem, we become overwhelmed.

But we've also seen that isolating problems in life – for example, trying to 'fix' a single risk without considering the further risks of doing so – can bring unimaginative, inadequate and often counter-productive results.

Do we have to remain stuck between a rock and hard place, or are there ways we can balance simplifying reality with recognising, and acting on, the vast, overlapping nature of the world?

What do we know? Assuming the examples in this book are true – which they do seem to be – then we know quite a lot. We know that nothing is really separate from everything else. We know that everything's connected in ways we can see but mostly in ways we can hardly fathom (there are at least 100 forces that cause tides, but they're invisible to all but a handful of experts – (148)). We know that everyone sees the world differently, and we know we mostly have to guess the ways others see it – certainly, if we really want to know how other people see the world we have to take a lot of time and trouble to explore. We know we label the world so as to make sense of it and we know that time and again our labels change. We know that the way we understand and communicate about the world changes partly because of us, not just because of it. We know that all experiences are a relationship between the information we receive and how we interpret it – there's no such thing as a pure experience that everyone has in exactly the same way.

We know that in every aspect of education, research and life in general we oversimplify (what you saw on last night's TV news is the perfect example of what we do). We know that people are deeply complex, and while we all share much about life and we are all similarly biological and psychological, we all have different histories, different stories, personal hopes and subjective fears. We know that values are not the solid, fixed entities we are told they are. We know – despite appearances – that there's no such thing as an isolated decision – all decisions emerge from a rich and complex background of social and physical reality. And we also know that when we try to change the world as if it is in separate pieces – by isolating and fixing THE cause of a problem – this works only for machines, not for human problems. We can fix a problem with a carburettor using a spanner, but we can't fix a problem with a village like this.

Because we know all this, if we want to act in the world with awareness, then we need to see past our simplifications to find ways that assist us to have richer interactions and to make deeply intelligent, sensitive decisions. The alternative is passive acceptance of what we're told, and unthinking adherence to rules and checkboxes that have been handed down to us, just because this is easier.

Consequently, the final chapter of this book offers a toolkit of practical approaches that anyone can use to improve their insight, awareness, questioning ability and their professional practice.

Toolkit Item One: Practice Mindful Labelling

The most important part of our toolkit – for health workers and for everyone else – is to learn to practice mindful labelling.

We have no choice but to label the world, but we do have a choice about how we do it. We can blindly accept our labels as true and right, or we can look critically at them, with the awareness that they are labels and not necessary truths. We can peel them back, look afresh at what's underneath them, and throw them away if it suits us.

Mindful labelling simply means using labels aware that they are labels. And the key to doing this well is to be continually aware of and open to the world's abundance.

Open Mindfulness

Just now I was walking Iggy in the local wood. It's summer as I write and the trees are in full leaf, and every sort of green you can imagine. It's tranquil in the wood, almost mystical in its deep beauty. If you allow it, the wood will gently dislodge your everyday worries. A respite from your pesky goblins, if you want it.

Feeling quietly peaceful I noticed some tall, purple foxgloves. They follow on from the bluebells in this wood, and in groups make a striking display. For some reason, I have no idea why, I walked over to one of the plants. I wanted to take a closer look at the flowers, which hang down at a slight angle from the stems, opening up from the bottom of the stem first, then over a few days turning to seed as the higher up flowers take their turn to bloom. The flowers are roughly the size of a child's thumb, and could be described as trumpet shaped, or like a windsock at an aerodrome, or if you stand them erect they could be a decorative mini-vase you could fill with water – vessels for more flowers still perhaps.

The open foxglove flowers form a convenient landing pad – similar to the mouth of a snapdragon flower – for insects who have only a short walk to the throat of the flower to gather the pollen. As a gardener I already knew all this – or at least I thought I did – and it would have been easy for me to walk on by. But my attention was caught by the white spots on the landing pad. They are small white circles, of subtly different sizes, each with the main purple of the flower in the centre. They look uncannily like small rain drops or dew drops, and I'm guessing – who really knows – that these too are an inducement to bees, which encyclopaedias tell me are the plants' chief pollinators.

Each flower is quite beautiful, but what struck me most was the pattern of the spots. I looked from one flower to the next and not one of the patterns was the same. Some of the flowers bore so many spots it looked like snow, others were more sparse, with fewer larger spots. Why, I wondered, does every flower have a different pattern? Why can't each flower have the same pattern, or why can't there be just a few standard patterns? Is every digitalis flower unique?

I don't know how to answer these questions and as far as I can research on the internet and in books, no-one else does either. There is some evidence – though this cannot be certain – that no snowflake is ever the same shape (144) but no-one knows about foxgloves.

This experience gives hope. We think we know so much but really we know very little – and the history of science tells us that most of what we think we know will in any case be proven to be false in the course of time (145). It also – I think – shows us what sort of toolkit we should be aiming for, both as health carers and just as thoughtful, curious human beings.

I saw the patterns on the foxgloves, and asked the question about their difference, because I had space. Because of the quiet wood I was able to open my mind and see the world just a little differently. I know reality is a relationship between me as a receiver and it as a source, and that it is therefore eternally elusive, but I do still have choices about how I look at it. And if I look at the external world – or myself or other people – with care – I can create a richer picture. I can – if I so choose – see some of the meadow beyond the goblins.

One way to describe my experience of the foxgloves is 'mindfulness', a well-known set of techniques meant to help people see beyond the stress and pressure of daily life:

> Mindfulness is a mental state achieved by focusing one's awareness on the present moment, while calmly acknowledging and accepting feelings, thoughts, and bodily sensations. By being fully present in this way – not forcing things or hiding from them, but actually being with them, we create space to respond in new ways to situations and make wise choices. We may not always have full control over our lives, but with mindfulness we can work with our minds and bodies, learning how to live with more appreciation and less anxiety. (146)

The techniques are simple enough, with practice, and include 'mindful observation', which is more or less what I was doing with the flowers. To achieve mindful observation, you should choose a natural object from within your immediate environment and focus on watching it for a minute or two – a flower or an insect, or even the clouds or the moon. All you need do is notice the thing you are looking at – relax into the object. Look at it as if you are seeing it for the first time. Or you could try 'mindful immersion': for example, if you are cleaning your house, you can pay attention to every detail of the activity. Rather than treat it as a regular chore, you can create a new experience by noticing every aspect of your actions: feel and become the motion when sweeping the floor, sense the muscles you use when scrubbing the dishes, develop a more efficient way of wiping the windows clean. The idea is to discover new experiences – create richer realities – within a familiar routine task (147).

I think, though, that mindfulness on its own is not enough for the toolkit. I think it's a good start, allowing us to see past our habitual views of life, but mindfulness doesn't ask questions. And since the toolkit is mostly meant to help health carers offer better health care, I think there has to be room for curiosity, intelligence, questioning and exploration. There has to be scope in the toolkit to create better understandings of the world around us. That has to be the point of it.

An example that shows the sort of approach I have in mind is offered by the author Hugh Aldersey-Williams, in his book *Tide: The Science and Lore of the Greatest Force on Earth* (148). Quite early in his book Aldersey-Williams describes a personal experiment that, before he did it, seemed a little bizarre even to him, such is our conditioning to accept the accounts of the world we are given in schools and in text books. His book is about tides, a natural force that influences us all one way or another. Most people think we understand tides, assuming that the schoolchild account that the moon's gravity pulls the water back and forth in a regular motion is true. But in fact this is not true at all – there is an incredible array of forces in play, if you care to look for them.

Aldersey-Williams admits 'it is an odd idea simply to sit and watch the water for twelve or thirteen unbroken hours', but that is what he chose to do, to try to get closer to the force that fascinates him, and to dispel the simplistic, unadventurous view by means of his personal journey. I think his is a perfect example of what every health worker – and every policymaker – should do. Don't take other people's word for it. Think for yourself. Observe for yourself. Ask your own questions. Challenge conventional answers – if they're conventional assume they are telling only part of the story, and indeed may be totally wrong.

Aldersey-Williams made his observations of the tide one warm September morning shortly after dawn, in fine weather. As a scientist he began to take readings of the depth of the water as the tide quickly began to ebb, flowing back toward the rest of the sea. He felt excitement in his voyage – he was not merely mindful but thoughtful too. He noticed turbulence around a bridge support which was creating a succession of small whirlpools, which he describes as 'commas and semi-colons swept away by the current'. Then he observed that the whirlpools were rotating both clockwise and anti-clockwise. He had no idea why. Probably no-one does because no-one has paid attention to this phenomenon, just as we neglect countless other phenomena we fail to see seriously.

Aldersey-Williams began to become inundated with questions, because his eyes were open, he wanted to see for himself, and he wanted to try to understand what he was witnessing in his own way. It seems to me that this is precisely what each of us should do as much as we possibly can, both in work and in our personal lives. This quote, I believe, should be an exemplar to us:

> The water here is so murky that I cannot tell how deep it is, and I cannot easily investigate one thing I wished to – how the tide flows at different depths. If I were to track a certain cubic centimetre of water from the top surface of the high tide, would it go down until it reached the bottom, or would it go out sideways? Down or out? We talk about the tide being in or out, but the level of the water goes up or down. Which is it? Or is it a combination of the two? And which water flows the fastest? The water on the surface where it meets less friction from the seabed? Or the momentous water in the bulk of the flow, at mid-depth? Does my imaginary volume of water retain its dimensions for long, or is it stretched out as it goes like a piece of bubblegum pulled from the teeth? Or does it spread more complicatedly, tangling hydra-like with similar briny cubic centimetres on all sides? Naïve questions perhaps, but I feel I should know. (148)

Perhaps they are naïve questions. Probably – possibly – oceanographers know the answers, but that depends on what they are interested in, what questions they ask, and whether or not they are content to accept received wisdom or think for themselves (google searches reveal that most oceanographers believe the moon is the main force behind tides, which Aldersey-Williams flatly denies). But whether they are naïve questions or not, they are Aldersey-Williams' questions and by asking them he not only begins to challenge established views, which may well be wrong, but he opens the door to deeper ways to appreciate the world around him – and surely this is a lesson we might all benefit from.

Rather remarkably, he also discovered that the tide does not, after all, ebb and flow in a steady way, at the same speed all the time. This is not intuitive, but it is something I've suspected for a long time, though never bothered to investigate. I feel I was wrong not to do so now (I lived for many years beside the sea in New Zealand). Time's short, I should have explored for myself – but for now I am content to listen to Aldersey-Williams' curiosity, since I am still on a journey of my own:

> By four, I am beginning to feel impatient. Far from being at one with the Zen of it all, I am wondering if the tide will ever return. It is now more than three hours past the moment mid-way between the two highs. What can explain this apparent irregularity? Is the tide not a well-oiled machine like a piston pumping …? Is this disturbance something that happens everywhere, or just here? Does it happen on every tide here, or just on some? What perturbation of the cosmic clockwork is this? (148)

I don't know. But I do know there is so much none of us understand, and I also know that we are equipped to understand more, if we really want to. And if we are health workers I think we should, because if we can see even a bit more clearly we are likely to be more helpful to others.

Mindful Labelling

There are countless examples of labelling in this book – much of it mindless rather than mindful. For example, values-based recruitment is mindless labelling, because 'values labels' obscure deeper truths and cannot operate as assumed. The 'four principles' approach to ethics is mindless labelling for the same reasons. Calling sensitive, intelligent beings 'livestock' is mindless labelling because it minimises reality and is designed to prevent thoughtful reflection. Calling a sick person who doesn't want to do what you want him to do 'difficult' or 'non-compliant' is mindless labelling, because there is so much more to the person hidden behind the label.

Mindless labelling attempts to make one possible way of viewing the world the only way to view it.

Mindful labelling is done for the opposite reason to mindless labelling. Mindful labelling makes suggestions, indicates connections, is always tentative and is meant to be thought about and acted on with caution. There are, for example, thoughtful psychiatrists who use the official set of diagnostic labels as a convenient way to communicate conditions to other health professionals and patients, but do not assume that these labels accurately reflect reality. There is the world of difference between saying 'you have explosive personality disorder' and 'some of your behaviours fit with an official category called explosive personality disorder, but there is clearly a lot more going on with your life than this'.

A mindless psychiatrist might say:

> … your child has attention deficient hyperactivity disorder, I will prescribe a drug to cure him …

whereas a mindful psychiatrist might say:

> … according to our manual of mental illnesses your child could be defined as ADHD, but it is very important to be aware that this is just one way to look at what is going on. We can use this label if you think it will be helpful, but we are not obliged to, even if he seems to fit every criteria in the book. ADHD was not even recognised as an illness until relatively recently, and you may not want your child labeled in this way. You may want to think about how all our behaviours are a result of complex factors both within us and external to us, and consider whether it is fair to place the entire responsibility for the problems you perceive on your son. Shall we discuss this and look at all the options we might pursue to help your child live a more fulfilling life?

I use labels as much as anyone else. As we saw earlier, I make distinctions in my theory of ethics, calling some situations 'dramatic' and others 'persisting'. I created an 'ethical grid' deliberately constructed of four separate layers (practicalities, consequences, duties and purpose) and twenty separate tiles people might use to understand a problematic situation and work out what to do. And I developed a way of thinking about health that suggests health carers should flesh out several categories – for instance, 'need', 'information' and 'education' – according to prevailing circumstances. What's more, I recommend using one very large label – 'create autonomy' – as shorthand, initial guidance in every health care situation.

However, all the labels I use are mindful – I was certainly mindful as I was creating them – and they are meant to be used mindfully. The labels I use are meant as indicators and possibilities, not as truths, and they are not meant to be seen as ultimately separate from each other. They are just a convenient way to express possible ways of thinking about things. They are all connected, and in a way they each contain all the others – they are each just starting points in a reflective process. For example, in one version of the ethical grid there is a tile labelled 'increase benefit for society', which is one consideration that some people might find helpful to add to the mix when deciding what to do in some situations. In using the ethical grid, the idea is that the person deliberating will first of all decide whether any particular tile is helpful, and if it is so judged will then balance that tile against other tiles, for example, 'evidence', 'risk', 'law', 'respect for others' and so on. After a while, with experience, the grid can be used with just the one tile – like 'increase benefit for society' – to begin with, since thinking about 'increasing benefit for society' will inevitably trigger thinking about the rest of the grid too.

An Exercise in Mindful Labelling: Thinking Carefully About Health Promotion

Public health professionals frequently claim to be promoting health in the 'best interests' of the public, but they rarely specifically define how they know what these 'best interests' are and they rarely explain why they in particular should have the power to initiate campaigns to promote them. For example, 'public health experts' have for many years fought against smoking, on the ground that it can shorten people's lives. But while this is sometimes true, selecting 'smoking' as 'public health enemy number one' has had many consequences that people with different priorities consider unhealthy. These include continually inflating the risks of smoking, stigmatising smokers, creating false understandings of addiction, raising taxation to such a level that low income smokers are damaged, and generally creating an illogical taboo.

In fact, smoking it is no different from other habits which are approved of in moderation by official public health figures. Just like the other habits – drinking alcohol, exercise, eating meat – sometimes smoking is bad for you and sometimes it is good for you.

CNN recently reported that of the 40.9 million smokers in the US only 60 per cent are dependent on nicotine (149). Why then is it in the public interest to prohibit this activity from the remaining 40 per cent? And on what grounds can it be argued that all tobacco use is definitely harmful?

If you create a monolithic myth that all smoking is evil then, as you label it, you lose sight of the many ways in which this is not true: you see all smokers as addicted, you see them as weak and in need of help – but you don't see the pleasure, the free choice and the social aspects that people actually enjoy.

Despite the facts quoted from CNN, almost everyone seems to accept that smoking is bad for health, as a matter of fact. But it isn't. It's all a matter of which label you choose to apply, and whether you do so mindlessly or mindfully.

This can actually be proved, as I did in another book a few years ago (4). I simply listed three different health promotion plans.

Below is Plan A – completely conventional health promotion.

Health Promotion Plan A

Health promoters should try to stop people smoking

Because:

- Smoking causes sickness and shortens lives.
- Smoking makes people unfit.
- The medical treatment of smoking-related disease is expensive. Where such disease is treated by publicly-funded medical services, smoking incurs financial cost to the state.
- Smoking leads to absenteeism and loss of productivity and so incurs further cost to the state.

- Smoking damages non-smokers, physically (through passive smoking) and economically (because of its cost to the state – a cost which is ultimately borne by the individual taxpayer).
- Smoking is unaesthetic (it stains) and unhygienic (it smells).

Health promoters should try to stop people smoking by means of one or more of the following methods:

- *Education* – smokers should be presented with comprehensive evidence about the damage they do to themselves and others, and be enabled to make fully informed choices.
- *Training* – stop-smoking techniques should be freely and liberally available wherever people smoke. People should be given every opportunity to change their behaviour.
- *Indoctrination* – anti-smoking propaganda should be widely distributed to counteract the marketing campaigns of the tobacco companies. It should be made plain that tobacco-related disease is to be feared (scary real life images should be used), and the huge profits that tobacco companies make as a result of their trade should be given maximum publicity – as black a picture as possible should be painted about the undesirable effects of smoking and the immorality of the tobacco industry.
- *Legislation* – tobacco advertising should be banned, tobacco products should be taxed at a very high rate, smoking in public should be forbidden, smokers should be forced to bear the cost of all medical treatments made necessary by their smoking, smokers should be separated from non-smokers wherever possible.
- *Prohibition* – smoking should be outlawed altogether.

And here is Plan B – completely unconventional health promotion.

Health Promotion Plan B

Health promoters should encourage people to smoke

Because:

- Smoking helps people cope with life.
- Promoting smoking will help the tobacco industry employ more people (it is well known that unemployment is a cause of ill-health).

- Smoking raises taxes which governments can elect to spend on health services.
- Smoking reduces the level of chronic sickness in the elderly population because smokers tend to die sooner than non-smokers. Promoting smoking will lower the cost to the state of geriatric care.
- Young people think smoking is cool – it makes them feel they belong, and a sense of belonging is very important for health.
- Smoking is enjoyable – most smokers get pleasure out of smoking.

Health promoters should encourage people to smoke by means of one or more of the following methods:

- *Campaigning for unrestricted advertising* – in a capitalist country it ought to be legal to advertise any product that it is legal to sell.
- *Comprehensive advice on how to get the very most enjoyment from cigarette smoking* – what to smoke, what strength cigarette is best in which circumstances, when to use a filter and when not, how to roll your own, what the optimum frequency should be (this advice should be based on detailed scientific research undertaken by health promoters).
- *Advertising widely the many mental and social benefits that smoking offers.*

Here is Plan C – even more unconventional health promotion.

Health Promotion Plan C

Health promoters should try to stop people playing rugby

Because:

- Rugby causes serious injury and shortens lives.
- Rugby makes people unfit.
- The medical treatment of rugby-related injury incurs considerable cost to the state.
- Rugby leads to absenteeism and loss of productivity, and so incurs further cost to the state.
- Rugby damages non-rugby players economically.
- Rugby is unaesthetic, it promotes aggression and venerates brawn over brain.

Health promoters should try to stop people playing rugby by means of one or more of the following methods:

- *Education* – rugby players should be presented with evidence of the damage they do to themselves and others, should be shown alternative leisure activities, and enabled to make fully informed choices about their behaviours free from social pressures.
- *Indoctrination* – anti-rugby propaganda should be widely distributed to counteract the marketing campaigns of the sportswear companies and brewers, glossy 'Stop Rugby' brochures should be distributed nationally, there should be a national 'no-rugby day' on a winter's Saturday, and terrifying advertisements showing ex-rugby players paralysed as a result of neck injuries should be aired repeatedly on TV.
- *Legislation* – there should be a ban on the advertising of rugby games, admission to rugby matches should be highly taxed, and so on.

The original intention in describing these three plans was to show that none of them is a neutral response to evidence, rather each is constructed according to this general formula:

$$\text{Various pieces of evidence} + \text{Various sorts of opinion} = \text{A health promotion plan}$$

And this means that they are all, equally morally controversial. *Plan A* merely seems uncontroversial because we are so used to it.

I offer these three plans now merely as an illustration of the difference between mindless and mindful labelling. Conventional, mindless labelling looks at the three plans and assumes that only *Plan A* is labelled correctly. Mindful labelling examines all three plans, recognising that they are all essentially of the same form, but with different judgements about what is important. Mindful labelling sees that the different labels challenge us and lead us to the only possible conclusion – that it is not reality, or neutral evidence, that drives health promotion, but deeper forces (political, ethical, self-interest, ignorance, stupidity and so on) that we can chose to go along with or fight against. It is up to us what labels we choose, after all.

Toolkit Item Two: Always Try to Understand Your Own and Other People's Decision Bubbles

The Official View of How We Make Decisions

There are many different versions of the Official View, but in essence it's that we make our decisions using evidence and logic to work out the most effective plan. This sort of decision making can be easily visualised. Just think of a single bubble. Let's call it a 'decision bubble'. Within the bubble there are all the steps of the plan – just think of any logical plan you have ever made and imagine it's inside the bubble (150).

Whatever plan you are thinking of, it will have certain form: it will have a goal or goals, it will have some strategy to achieve the goal and some means of delivering the strategy. For example, your plan might be to buy an ice cream – in which case 'buying an ice cream' is your goal, 'finding the nearest retail outlet and ordering the ice cream' is your strategy and 'asking for the ice cream and paying for it' is your means.

Any logical plan can be visualised within the single bubble, without exception. Obviously some logical bubbles are extraordinarily complicated. Think for instance about what deciding to gain a PhD might involve for a school student just completing her school qualification. This plan must involve very many different goals, strategies and means, as well as even more factors beyond her control. But nevertheless it could fit into a decision bubble: if I want to achieve a PhD then, from here, I must also apply to a university, choose a subject I am good at, be accepted by the university, enrol in the programme, find out where the lectures are held … and so on and so forth.

If you like, you can think of the PhD plan as lots of little plans in lots of little bubbles, all of them logically connected within a much bigger decision bubble. The crucial thing about the whole decision bubble plan is that it needs to be logical and practical to stand a chance of working. If you managed no passes in your school qualification exams, or if you have no chance of paying for your university course, or if you want to do a subject you are useless at then your decision bubble would be irrational.

But – and this is crucial – while the plan has to make sense, this is not the most interesting thing about decision bubbles.

Because we make so many decisions in our lives we actually do see them as bubbles, popping into and out of existence as the need arises and as decisions are made and time moves on. And because we are used to so many decision bubbles every day, we tend to see them as spontaneously generated: 'you know what, I think I'll go ride my bike for half an hour …' It's as if decision bubbles just spring to life out of thin air.

But of course they don't. Every decision bubble, no matter how small and transient, is formed out of a sea of influences we are mostly unaware of: our personalities, our histories, our environment, our values – and all these change too. If we want to practice thoughtful health care, then we must always try to see both the logical bubble and what has brought it into existence.

We can choose to see other people and their decisions as complex and multifactorial, or we can see them as stupid and thick, and everything in between. But what is certain is that there are reasons for their choices that if we and they can comprehend them even just a little better, will help us

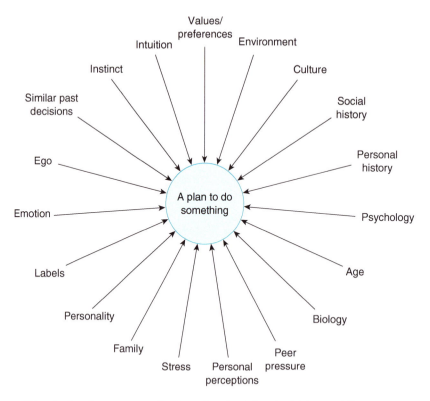

Figure 8.1   A simple representation of a decision bubble, and its causes

appreciate them more deeply. We do not have to agree with their decision bubbles just because we may understand their causes a little better. We don't have to respect them either. But we can look at them with more awareness, and maybe a little more sympathy.

Why would I decide to ride my bike? We might suppose it's just out of habit, but that would miss the ever-present deeper reasons, many of which we can only guess, but which must be there: I want to stay fit; I get a buzz from the wind in my hair; I want my legs to stay strong; I need some space; I like the wild animals I see on my favourite ride; I am procrastinating; it's an excuse to ride to the pub; I like being solitary sometimes (and there must be a further sea of reasons for this); it calms me down; it frees my mind; it's a bit risky; it's a timeless thing to do and it makes me forget how old I am; I have the choice; I have some control on my bike; it helps me forget everything that upsets me, and everything I have done wrong.

Our Decisions are Not Separate

We have already seen – from Russell's explanation of appearance and reality in Chapter 3 – that in a way we are separate from each other, since we all experience the world physically, emotionally and historically in unique ways. How I view this school, or this car, or this person is not the way you see these things, it cannot be how you view these things, because no-one else has your perspective. We also know, thanks to the efforts of many academic disciplines, that we construct reality. We don't receive the world as empty vessels, rather we build what we think the world is by combining the information we receive – sounds, colours, touch, words, orders from authority, the law, love, violence – everything – with the manner in which we receive it. To a short-sighted person a seascape is not at all the same as it is to a person with 20/20 vision. To a deaf person music is either nothing, or experienced as if in a different dimension (151) from music heard by a person with statistically normal hearing. To a Christian death is a 'passing' whereas to an atheist it's a finality – which means that at a funeral of a friend the Christian and the atheist will have at least some different perceptions, even if they are unaware of them.

So, yes, in a way life is a lonely vigil, a perplexion from which we depart entirely on our own – after all, no-one else experiences our death. And yet there are far deeper connections that show – whether we like it or not – that we are not separate at all, but part of a deeply connected environment (it's impossible to find the right word to define this richness) where we're not really the autonomous individuals we think we are. As we've seen, we find it very hard to see this deeper world because of our sense that we're separate islands of existence, and because of our system of labelling everything in chunks. But this is really nothing more than a habit.

Right now I'm sitting in my garden. I can see a wall, a pergola, a mirror, poppies, strawberries, cornflowers; I can hear birds singing and, in the distance, cars passing. I've gardened for many years so I know a lot about each individual plant. My strawberries are in hanging baskets and they are putting out tendrils. I know these tendrils are 'runners' – shoots meant to contact the earth and root in order to make new plants. So in a way, I not only see the strawberries I see separate bits of them, but an inexperienced gardener is likely to see only the one plant. In fact, there's a fuchsia in the basket as well – two separate species in combination. But it's likely that a non-gardener will see only the one plant. And it's just as possible that a child, or a person passing overhead in a balloon or hang-glider, or a photographer, or a painter would either unconsciously, or through choice, see a whole garden: not separate bits but a single whole garden.

Because we can choose to see things in whatever size separate bits we like – from atoms and electrons to a single universe – I believe that essentially everything is connected. It's we who make the disconnections, and it's we who so frequently suffer emptiness, meaninglessness and isolation as a consequence.

About an hour ago I was walking in a leafy, early summer wood with Iggy. I never feel solitary in a wood, even when I'm alone. Everything seems connected – a complex, intricate whole – and I feel connected to everything too. It's an intensely comforting feeling. It relaxes me, and then thoughts, ideas, memories flow into me (or flow out of me, I don't think it much matters which way round it is). Mostly I think of my father, who seems to visit my consciousness when I am wrapped up in mysterious pathways, crunching sticks, leaves, dappled sunlight and all the smells of the damp earth. Today, I was wondering what he'd think of my life, and whether he watches me. I imagined he might have mixed feelings. I felt a little rueful, but laughed it off and began to wonder how I got here – how any of us get where we are.

It's tempting to think of ourselves as in control, to think that when we make decisions it is each of us, alone, who do so. But if everything really is connected then this belief is undoubtedly a delusion.

Tracing a few steps in my life, I came to the rather obvious conclusion that if it had not been for my father's illness, not only would I not be in this wood, with this dog, and with these memories, I would be a different person altogether. Some parts of me are pre-determined. I'd probably look more or less the same, have the same IQ and basic biological and psychological make-up – but the rest of me would be different: not because of me as a separate individual, but because my external environment (if that is the right expression) would be different. Had my father not been ill I would not have been expelled from school, I would not have been so confused and lost as an adolescent, I would not (I think) have been so reckless with my life, I would not have read the escapist books I read, I would not have seen myself (then) as so separate and apart from everything else, and I think I would not have had some of the friends I had back then. And of course, it's not just the personal things that would not be as they are now – I would have gone to a different school, I would have lived somewhere else (my parents told me they would have moved for sure), I would have had different teachers, heard different stories, come across different opportunities. Almost everything would be different, as it would be for all of us. The briefest glance from a passing stranger is enough to change the course of history.

Just about all of the forces that design our lives are unseen by us, until we start to look seriously at them. And – amongst oceans of puzzling implications – this most definitely includes how we make our decisions. We do not make decisions in isolation. We make them as connected beings, and we do not really understand how or why we make them.

There are, of course, many people who claim to know exactly how we make decisions. Economists say we calculate what to do in order to maximise the consequences in our own best interests. Psychologists say we decide according to personality type and peer pressure. Some misguided 'ethicists' say we decide according to ethical rules and principles. Biologists say that many of our decisions are instinctive, reflex actions that build up over time to create personal patterns of decision making. And many neuroscientists say we decide not just with our brains but with our physical senses. For example, a blush is not just a blush, it's an involuntary driver of our behaviour.

I'm sure each of these outlooks is partly correct, as we can all see by thinking about how we make our own decisions. But I'm equally sure that even taken together, they do not tell the whole story. The world is so much more of an enigma than we're prepared to countenance. If we are to grow more civilised and if we are to be more helpful to others, it is vital that we understand this.

How do I know this? Well, I don't. It's speculation, but I think it's at least plausible. My most compelling personal example of the unseen forces that underlie our decision making also concerns my father, in a subtle way. In my final year as a post-graduate at university I needed to work out what I was going to do next, and I began to find myself increasingly in the medical school library – not reading much clinical material but exploring books on the philosophy and sociology of medicine. I was finishing my PhD on 'rationality' – which was about how our decisions cannot be purely logical and systematic (30-plus years ago, my goodness). I was becoming more and more interested in health and medicine. Once I was awarded the degree my interest in health blossomed further, and I ended up with a job as a Research Assistant looking into nurses' conceptions of health, and I began to write a book originally called *What is Health?* (2).

Why I was pursuing this route was completely obscure to me. I seemed to be on an interesting path – maybe influenced by a course I did in the philosophy of science in my third year taught by a lecturer I admired. But otherwise I assumed this to be nothing more than random, just the way things turned out.

One day I was explaining what I was up to to a friend, who knew me fairly well. When I said I had no idea why I was doing this or where it was leading she burst out laughing.

'Really David? Are you serious?' she asked.

'What do you mean?' I was genuinely baffled.

'You mean you really don't know?'

'I have no idea.'

'It's because of your Dad and all your experiences. Of course you are going to be interested in medicine and illness and disability and – the opposite side to this, aren't you? It's no secret why you want to think and write about health. It's what your life has been about so far,' she smiled kindly.

I was shocked. Put like that it really was obvious – what else would it be about? But I had no idea. I also had no idea how many of the millions of other decisions that led up to deciding to write about health had been based on my profound reaction to my father's Multiple Sclerosis. In order to get to a place where I was intellectually and emotionally equipped even to consider creating a theory of health I had made literally countless decisions that at the time were equally beyond my comprehension, but after my friend's revelation they became alarmingly explicable. Choosing to go to university, studying philosophy, studying sociology, choosing thoughtful friends, choosing particular courses to study, rejecting so much of what I was taught in order to go what I thought was my own way. Was I really on a path to here all along, making exactly the decisions that would get me exactly here? Could I really have been so deliberate while being so utterly unaware? I don't know how to answer these questions, but it does seem like a great many of my apparently chance choices were in some unperceived way worked out by me, or perhaps for me. I don't know.

But I do know that my decisions were clearly not rational in the conventional sense. I did not articulate my reasoning, I did not knowingly balance my options, I was not explicitly following my own best interests. I was certainly making decisions, but these were mostly motivated by unseen forces, and I think it is this way for all of us.

This is why it's best to try to see as many connections as we can, as often as we can. And this is why it's best to think of decisions as bubbles, but not separate ones. Decision bubbles are only fleetingly separate – they emerge from a mix of circumstances that are beyond our comprehension, and merge back into them, minutely adding to them, once they are made.

Toolkit Item Three: Understand That Work for Health is Work to Create Autonomy

Chapter 5 introduced the importance of creating autonomy, and explained how it might be done. Here's a further worked example, to reinforce the idea.

Helping Catherine

We first met Catherine when she was alienated and scared, walking overwhelmed along a hospital corridor, after being told she had Alzheimer's

Disease. We also debated what should happen to Petra, Catherine's dog. Now Catherine is in a rest home. Most of the day she sits silently, withdrawn and morose. This is not unusual for people with Catherine's diagnosis, so it can be tempting just to leave her be, and get on with working with more responsive patients. But this is not the point of working for health. Working for health requires thoughtful observation and the recognition that every person, no matter what their present situation, has positive potentials that could, if released, enhance their lives.

If it is to be fulfilling, life requires our attention. I'm looking at some poppies in my garden right now, but I am distracted. My attention is on too much at once. I'm thinking about an appointment I cancelled, which will probably not be well-received. I'm wondering if my partner is happy. I'm thinking I need to catch a train tomorrow morning. I'm unsure if this book I'm writing is any good. I'm hot and I feel I need some air.

I stopped the noise in my thoughts, deliberately. I went back to looking at the poppies, calmly and quietly, giving them proper attention.

The poppies are in a plastic wall box. They are so heavy the box is pulling away from the wall. The leaves are hanging down as if they will cascade from the box at any moment. The flowers are yellow and orange. There is one white one too.

The longer I look the more comes into view. The tendrils of the strawberry plant in the hanging basket above them have reached down, as if to touch the poppies. The tendrils are swaying and each poppy flower is moving, mostly from side to side but one is spinning in a circle. Everything is motion. It's quite a dance.

Now I can see the bees too. As they arrive the flowers move more quickly, as if beckoning the bees. Surely that is just my fantasy, but by paying attention I allow the thoughts to come, and I see so much more. I had no idea how much my poppies twirled. It's such a show, and it's changed my mind.

We should try to see Catherine as if she's a poppy, despite the likelihood that by quietly watching her other people will think we are being lazy.

We know that a large part of every decision and every action is not conscious but comes about through unseen forces that we do not need to articulate. So we can be a witness to Catherine's choices, even if she is mentally unaware she is making them.

Just now, Catherine had a bowl of cornflakes, which she had chosen from other cereal options offered to her. We know that even a decision to have a bowl of cornflakes – as simple as it appears – comes out of a rich bed of history, emotion, memory, knowledge and so on. The decision to have cornflakes is never just random and never just logic.

This may seem trivial, but it isn't if you want to work for Catherine's health. Look closely at her, there may be a way to create more autonomy. Look and see what there is.

Catherine loves cornflakes, that's clear. She likes warm milk better than cold, and she likes a lot of sugar on her cornflakes. You notice that for some reason eating cornflakes helps Catherine feel less scared and anxious – you know she is afraid because her body is tense and she clearly hates not knowing where she is.

Whenever Catherine is eating cornflakes she likes to have you sit with her, and sometimes she will talk. She will talk about her dog and about her children, not always in the present but you can see it makes her happy. Today, by surprise, her daughter is here as Catherine is eating her cornflakes. For some reason Catherine seems to recognise her daughter in the present, and is communicating positively with her body and some words.

It is as if cornflakes open a door for Catherine, and therefore for you. Thinking about cornflakes – and the decision bubbles that lead up to Catherine eating them – is an important therapeutic opportunity if you want to take it. You may be able to use what you have observed about Catherine and cornflakes to create more autonomy – isn't this what health work should be all about?

Toolkit Item Four: Use Connected Frameworks to Guide Your Thought and Practice

Chapter 5 briefly explained the background to the Foundations Template, which is fully explained in *Health: The Foundations for Achievement* (2), which can be specified in as much practical detail as necessary, in order to create thoughtful care for every patient. There are many other frameworks you might also choose, especially in the nursing literature. Typically, these frameworks ask you to define the problem, consider your options, reflect on them, put what you decide into action and then reflect some more (152).

Some are quite detailed, but it is better that they are not, since in the end each health worker must observe, think and act for herself.

As mentioned earlier, in other books I have offered a connected framework for thinking called the ethical grid (105), a diluted version of which is part of the Think Screen you can explore in some of the cases used in this book's Values Exchange. The grid is meant to suggest lots of options to you to help you deliberate thoroughly in every situation. What are the practicalities? What consequences matter most? Do you have ethical obligations? How do you see your purpose in this particular situation?

The grid exemplifies the sort of framework I recommend. It is broad and has lots of different ideas in it, but nothing is concrete. There are no rules. No checklists. Just options you can consider if you want, in the context you are thinking and working in.

How you conceive of the Foundations Template, or ethical grid, or any similar sort of tool, is absolutely crucial. Like everything else that can be spelled out, you can use it bit by bit, according to instructions, in a set way that is likely to work in some circumstances. But if you do it this way, you risk getting stuck in just that one way of thinking. It's much better to throw it away from time to time, and find another way. Show it to colleagues, friends, your clients – ask them how they would design a holistic template – and learn from that. Have a conversation with others – tell them what's worked for you and then ask them how it could be done better.

Toolkit Item Five: Work Out What you are committed to and Act on it

You can call this 'working out what you value', 'deciding your ethical outlook' or 'telling right from wrong', but these are just labels. It doesn't matter what you call your commitment in the end. The point is to work out – and always be prepared to revise – where you stand in life. In particular – and this is obviously central if you are a health worker – work out where you stand in relation to other people. And be honest as you do so, it is so easy for us to deceive ourselves.

There is definitely a need for caution. It is easy to cite official slogans, like 'putting the patient first', and claim to be committed to them. But are you really? Be honest – what do you really value? Go on to the Values Exchange and respond to situations that make you uncomfortable. What does this tell you?

Certainly, the evidence from the Values Exchange is overpoweringly that most health professionals do not put the patient first. Most definitely do not support patients to achieve what the patients say are in their 'best interests'. Below is an example you can respond to in order to see this for yourself.

Emily Smith (57) (not her real name) was a hugely popular singer in the 1980s, making a string of hit songs, and a small fortune in the process. Her career peaked in the early 90s, and then plummeted, leaving her confused, depressed and a heavy drinker. Emily has received psychiatric treatment (including voluntary rehabilitation and two compulsory detentions for her own safety, for detox) intermittently ever since.

Seven years ago Emily received a liver transplant, amid much publicity. The transplant was successful, and Emily thrived for three years. She stopped drinking entirely and re-launched her career, with moderate success.

For the last 18 months, again under a media spotlight and unconfirmed rumours that she is again drinking heavily, Emily's transplant has begun to fail.

Emily's medical team has agreed to offer a fresh transplant, but under the clear condition that she drinks no alcohol until the operation, and never drinks again afterwards.

By coincidence, you are driving home from work and notice the car in front moving erratically. After five minutes or so, the car pulls up, mounting a kerb in the process. As a health professional you are concerned for the health and safety of the driver, and park behind the car.

You move to the driver's door and see a middle-aged woman slumped over the wheel. You bend down to examine her and immediately smell alcohol strongly on her breath. You ask her if she is OK and she rallies, nodding her head and looking up at you.

You are surprised to see that it is unmistakeably Emily Smith.

She says, 'I'm OK now thanks,' and gets out of the car. 'It's my flat up there – I'm OK.' She then walks unsteadily up the steps, and eventually succeeds in entering her flat.

What should you do? You could have called the police but since Emily is now in her flat you dismiss this thought.

However, like most of the population, you are aware that Emily's liver transplant depends on her sobriety.

What should you do? What are the considerations? Is there an ethical thing to do?

It is proposed that as a health professional, you report this incident to her medical team.

Add your response on the Values Exchange: http://thoughtful.vxcommunity.com/Issue/think-stop-eighteen-right-to-drink/12346

You can see the general results before you begin. They make a startling pattern. Where the patient is seen to be doing something risky to themselves, between 85 and 100 per cent of health professional respondents will try to stop them, even if the patient is expressing a clear and informed preference to engage in the risky behaviour.

This is no small finding. The NHS Constitution tells us that everyone in the health service:

> … should support individuals to promote and manage their own health. NHS services must reflect, and should be coordinated around and tailored to, the needs and preferences of patients, their families and their carers. (17)

But as a matter of fact most NHS workers will mostly not do this. Emily Smith's preference is to be left alone and, as far as we know, to receive a liver transplant. Rachel's preference is to end her life, with sympathy and support, since she finds her burns and amputated legs unbearable. But the great majority of respondents will not support the choices of patients like Emily and Rachel, whatever the Constitution says, and usually whatever they say too.

Officially, NHS staff are supposed to follow the Constitution, as vague as it is. But they do not always do so. They follow their own stars, many preferring to avoid personal risk and many others making strikingly paternalistic judgements about what patients deserve – about 30 per cent of respondents think other people are more deserving of the liver transplant, based on the scantiest evidence about Emily the rock singer, and no evidence at all about any other potential recipient of a liver.

At the very least, this should give the respondents – and the rest of us too – pause for thought. We already know that pressure to follow 'official values' cannot deliver (see Chapter 1). So in fact rather than follow codes and policy, people have to decide for themselves, based on multiple factors, mostly unseen by them. The question is: on what basis are they deciding and how deeply are they thinking? On what basis do you decide and how deeply do you think? What are you committed to?

The evidence, from Values Exchange data, is that the bulk of respondents are not accustomed to reflecting about their commitments in general or their purposes at work. Instead most offer 'gut reactions', which are not examined in depth. Values Exchange respondents are encouraged to use philosophical and practical concepts to help their deliberations, but they mostly just say straight out what they think, like comment threads in newspapers rather than reflective, self-aware analysis. There are exceptions, but most people on the Values Exchange fire from the hip.

We Need to Build a Thoughtful Culture

This is hardly an ideal situation. If it is to improve then two changes are required. The first is to alter the 'official focus', changing it from the totally unrealistic command culture which insists 'you will always conform to the Constitution', 'you will abide by these values', 'you will meet everybody's needs simultaneously', to a culture of reflection, self-awareness, personal responsibility and commitment. The second is to stop worrying about recruiting people with 'the right values' and start thinking about offering all students and staff an education which equips them – and gives them permission – to think for themselves, to question authority, to challenge received wisdom, to find creative solutions to daily problems, to work together thoughtfully and kindly, to feel free to speak their minds and listen to others doing the same, without fear. In short, the aim must be to create and sustain a culture which gives health professionals the space to think, to debrief and feedback continually, and to consult and work with patients and other carers as a matter of course.

I'm afraid that seasoned health professionals will look at these two changes and at best think they are idealistic, and at worst think I'm nuts for even suggesting such a cultural shift might be possible. Yet if systemic reform – which so many official reviews recommend – is ever to come about we need to take it seriously. Systemic change will not happen if bits and pieces of the system are fiddled with separately. It can only happen holistically, which means enabling every member of staff to be constantly reflective about everything around them, and offering a critical education as standard to every health professional student. Of course they need to learn clinical skills, but just as much they need to learn philosophy, politics, psychology and social science – in a deeply connected way, continually reinforced and with endless practical examples of how they might deal with personally and professionally challenging situations (whistle-blowing, for instance (153)). They need these tools to support their thinking and practice just as much as they need to know how to take blood pressure, give safe injections and insert a catheter.

They also need an enabling working environment in place. Systematic change must involve the whole picture. It's no good, for example, fostering personal reflection and a deeply connected education, if the system in practice is set against it. If health workers are to advocate for patients then everyone needs to have thought seriously about what advocacy means; whether you can disagree with a patient's goals and still advocate for them; whether you can advocate for patients who have competing needs (both needing a scarce therapy that only one can have); the extent to which external clinical factors affect advocacy (say the evidence is uncertain, or the patient misunderstands the evidence); whether you can advocate one thing for one patient and a conflicting thing for another; whether you can advocate for a patient if it seems not to fit with a code of some kind; and whether you can advocate for a patient if your boss tells you not to.

As the *Theory and Practice of Nursing* says:

> Sutor (1993) argues that patient advocacy is an impossible goal until it is enshrined within a legal framework which protects both nurses and their clients from possible sanctions from their employers. Nurses have learnt, sadly to their own cost, that there is a price to pay for speaking up for their clients. (154)

Without the space and time to think, it is a very big ask to expect every health worker to be clear about her ethical commitment.

What are you Committed to?

At the personal level, every health worker needs to be able to work out their 'moral commitment'. Everyone needs to have as good an idea as they can about where they stand ethically, and that requires being as clear as possible about their purpose – in life in general and as a paid health worker.

In contrast to the ubiquitous establishment view that there are right and wrong values, correct principles and objective moral truths, I believe (and have argued many times in print) that there are no moral standards beyond the human world. Just as we label everything else, so we label our behaviours. We invent ethics, it does not exist apart from us.

This does not mean that anything goes or that all behaviours are equally OK. It just means that no-one can prove 'ethical truth'. Instead, we must all decide what 'moral commitment' means to each of us, individually. And in health care this means that we have to have a theory about what we are doing and what is most important in our work – and as we have seen, any help with this is currently sadly lacking, and so by default most of us accept that fighting disease is an overriding priority. But this is mindless, not mindful.

Ethics is everywhere, not in separate chunks. Any actions made by competent human beings have the potential to affect others for better or worse. This is just obvious. Ethics is not a specialist discipline; it is the stuff of all our lives.

Because we live with others we constantly encounter ethical situations, whether or not we perceive them as such. Being pleasant, unpleasant (or anything else) to people during a Saturday morning trip around the supermarket are ethical actions – regardless of intent – because they have the potential to produce different sorts of meaningful consequences.

The task for anyone who wishes to be ethical is first to work out what 'being ethical' means, and then to devise the most effective strategies to achieve it. Since the founding question of ethics is 'how should I conduct my life in the presence of other lives?', the ethical challenge – at any time and in any place – is to work out what commitment to living to make.

My personal commitment starts with 'creating autonomy', and with working out how best to do this, and then acting. I most definitely fail to achieve this much more often than not, but at least I am aware of my failings. The fact that I am committed to creating autonomy at least means that I can be aware of all the times I don't live up to my commitment, and it means that if I want to I can always learn and try to do better next time.

Toolkit Item Six: Remember That Culture Change is Possible

The biggest barrier is not the size of the problem – though it is massive enough – but its nature. Without a thought-through understanding of the point of health care, there can be no systemic reform. It will always be piecemeal, no matter how many pieces you try to change.

Francis recommended nearly 300 specific changes, but while it seems logical enough to do this if you have identified so much that is wrong, in the end it merely fosters the packet trap. Fix this, fiddle with this, replace this bit, get some new nuts and bolts, make sure you go through a check list every hour for every patient, appoint right-thinking people – and the culture will be transformed. But it won't be. Bits of it may change a little, for a while, but they will inevitably be modified and absorbed into 'the way we normally do things around here'. A piecemeal reformer is like a person in quicksand: the more she tries to escape it the more it sucks her in.

For example, there are initiatives to change NHS culture to one where patients are part of the decision-making process, but so entrenched is the view that the patients are the recipients of therapy rather than participants in their care, that there is sustained resistance to this change:

> Clinicians are most likely to support those aspects of self-management that relate to a patient making behaviour and lifestyle changes in accordance with clinical advice. They are less likely to support people making independent judgements and taking independent actions when caring for themselves at home … They are least likely to support people being independent seekers of information. (155)

There are repeated pleas and attempts to involve patients more equally in their care, but this seems almost impossibly hard to do in any extended manner:

> There was overall agreement that co-production was about a new set of relationships with patients, new forms of practice from clinicians, and new forms of organisational change … (but) … co-production continues to be the exception rather than the norm, isolated to small pockets of practice … (we need to) … work … with clinicians to engage with how they think and feel (and introduce) … tools, methods, and strategies to shape practice and organisational culture. (156)

But:

> Despite the original visionary nature of the legislation, implementation has suffered through a prevailing culture of paternalism which puts risk aversion before individual rights … if vulnerable people

with compromised capacity are to achieve equal citizenship and their autonomous wishes are to be respected, they ought to be allowed to take risks, make mistakes, experiment and change course in their lives, just like every other citizen. (157)

Here is what one intelligent, insightful, retired nurse told me, reported verbatim:

> Nurses don't always understand that capacity is decision specific … And fluctuates … So what they have to do is know the person well enough to know when they are lucid … For example they will go in and turn a patient with dementia and not even ask if they want to be turned. Assuming they don't have capacity for any decision … Like the man I looked after … who wanted to watch the cricket … They turned him away from the television … He was terminal … I said he doesn't want to be turned he wants to watch the cricket … But they turned him … So I turned the bed around in the room so he could watch the cricket. But they didn't like that … because it looked scruffy …Well I said …that's what he wants … Leave him alone poor man … At handover time … they say he gets awful stroppy … I said I would if it was me I don't blame him … People fiddling with him every hour … And despite all the fiddling no one even noticed he was probably in kidney failure because they were so obsessed with Intentional Rounding and turning …

> Well the Mental Capacity Act 2005 came to turn around the paternalistic culture … In reality … practitioners don't always know how to apply it … And don't very often … because the policies are all so paternalistic – like Intentional Rounding and so on … which is meant to ensure standardised care for all but often has the negative effect of hiding people's individuality….. And there is the fear of being sued … They are too risk averse to implement it properly – nurse knows best – despite legislation designed to put patient preference first … And of course the policies conflict with each other too … And no one has the freedom, courage or motivation to challenge the policies or deviate or individualise policy to their own clinical area or specific patient needs…. the trouble is the whole hospital has a blanket top-down approach which is audited regularly by ward managers to ensure 'clinical dashboard targets'

reflect 'excellence'… but with so much inspection this culture induces fear, compliance and automated behaviours …. so it reduces the capacity for meaningful and critical engagement with each different patient … and then staff moan when they get policy top down when it should be bottom up … Yet they do nothing about it …

There are negative connotations associated with policy deviation … You are seen as potentially reckless … Yet really it is intelligent creativity … if it is person centred and you can justify it … Like the man watching the cricket … I would say he does not want to be turned … They would say he has had morphine he is confused he has brain mets … I would say he clearly says he wants to watch the cricket … That is good enough for me … And document it … It's not rocket science … Then they said he had morphine he has a bad headache … I said he has a headache because he is in renal failure and no one has made sure he drank the drinks you gave him … You have written on his fluid chart that you gave him fluid … But you didn't write that he didn't drink it … So his fluid chart is not accurate … Look at his output … 30 mls in 8 hours… Should be 30 mls at least an hour… All he needs is an IV infusion and he will be less confused which he will be if he is dehydrated … He wants to drink but he can't do it … But they say he is dying – he doesn't need an IV infusion … I said he does if he wants to drink and he has pain from dehydration …

(As told to me by Vanessa Peutherer, VX Learning Facilitator.)

Creating Autonomy Should Be at the Heart of Everything

How do we change wholeheartedly from a packet trap culture into an intelligent, creative, fearless culture? In a way it is very simple. Place 'creating autonomy' at the centre of everything that is done, from day one of health student education to every policy change and new plan.

Francis didn't need to list all those reforms. He just needed one: be crystal clear that the purpose of health care is first to 'create autonomy' in everyone in it, including every patient, every carer and every member of staff or volunteer. The purpose of the NHS must be – and must be seen to be – to enable people as complex, whole beings existing in an impossibly complicated reality to achieve as much of their positive potentials as possible. This should be the official ethos because it is meaningful, substantial and can be delivered in sensible, consistent practical ways. Make this the rationale of all health student education. Instil the ethos by encouraging creative thinking, self-awareness and a habit of questioning and challenging everything. Stop adding rules and commands on top of rules and commands. Help everyone to be prepared to go against the tide. Reward any initiative that supports freedom and creativity, even if it is against current policy.

Sustained clarity of purpose can change cultures.

Toolkit Item Seven: Remember That it is Up to you Whether you See Things as Separate or Connected

We know, from everything we have witnessed in this book, that the way we understand the world is not just to do with reality outside us. It is always a relationship between external factors – objects and events that are happening independent of us – and our perceptions of these external factors. This means that the world must appear different to each of us. It also means that once we are aware that this is the case, we can make conscious choices about how we want to see it, which is quite a gift.

It means that we do not have to feel totally controlled by external forces, because in truth we are not. We do not have to see the world always as a scientist might see it, or always as a priest might see it, or always as the rule book says it is, or always as your boss or your partner might see it. Our knowledge that reality is a relationship, not a given, really does offer us opportunity and power.

If we want to we can focus solely on the results of Farooq's latest blood analysis, and sometimes this will be the most creative and useful choice. And if we want to we can sit with Farooq for as long as we like, talking with him about his religion. We can do this if we have in mind that in the end all we want to achieve is a little more autonomy, a little more understanding, a little more possibility – just a little more movement in life for as many of us as possible.

Most of the time we all fail in this. We sit miserably in traffic queues on the way to work we don't want to do. We get frustrated and angry with stuff we will have forgotten next week. We see other people simplistically, as caricatures or cartoons of our own making. We try to control what we cannot possibly control – we fight snappy little goblins while the meadow sits serenely, waiting for us to contribute positively to it.

If we choose to be thoughtful we can have at least some grip on life's cliff face. We can see things as separate or as connected. We have that power.

The Calm Sea and the Tanker

There are so many examples that illustrate connectedness and our habitual denial of it – this book is crammed full of them. They're all worth including since we are so inclined towards delusion. I experienced one recently, during a midsummer's night in New Zealand.

I was sitting outside at a table in the late evening, overlooking a sea so calm it looked like mirror glass. The sea was gently illuminated by occasional street lighting, and was reflecting reds, oranges and mellow white from a distant road across the bay. I was doing little more than letting the experience wash over me, letting it cleanse me of a hectic day.

Then I noticed the sea had changed. Waves were rolling ashore, in a regular pattern, as if someone had pressed a button on a wave machine at a leisure centre. I thought nothing of it at first, but mentioned the change to my friend, who asked what I thought had caused this. I began to muse, thinking nonsense actually – thinking about the wind and the moon pulling the water – then the waves began to subside, the mirror sea returned and my mind emptied once more.

Then it happened again. This time I looked up to see a large tanker moving swiftly towards the nearby harbour. The waves were its wake. There were so many of them and they kept coming. It was several minutes before they subsided.

The night was otherwise so peaceful that it was tempting to feel annoyed at the boat for disrupting the blissful scene – to see the boat as an alien object that had unsettled the sea. Yet it dawned on me – vividly – that this is just one way of looking at the scene, not the absolutely true way.

I was looking at the boat as an object and the sea as a separate backcloth, but nothing in the nature of the scene meant that this is the way I must see it. Seeing the boat as a separate object was merely my interpretation.

Possibly because I was so relaxed, I was able to shift my perception. From my changed perspective, the boat was no longer a separate object but a connected part of the whole reality. The boat was not causing the waves – the boat and the waves were a part of the whole. There could be no waves without the boat and equally there could be no boat without the waves. This way of seeing was organic – like a poem with many related meanings – rather than separate objects awkwardly colliding.

The Sun and the Tree

Find a tree and look at it. At first sight it appears to be a unique, individual plant, standing alone, in competition with other nearby trees. And in a way it is, but in another way it isn't.

No tree can actually stand alone. Every tree is connected to everything else, as we all are. Its roots reach into the earth. It seeks water and sustenance that may have come from thousands of miles away, and which was itself generated by clouds and storms and seas equally far away. And beyond this, there's the sun, apparently 92,000,000 miles detached. What could be more separate than a distant sun and a tree?

And yet the sun reaches us, it feeds us, it warms us, and it feeds and warms the tree. The sun gives life to the tree and the tree gives life to the sun, by turning the sun's energy into a life force – by giving the sun a reason to shine. And this isn't separate. This is connected. Fundamentally, intimately connected. It's possible to see the sun and the tree as the same thing.

I am hardly the first person to appreciate the connectedness of the world, but it's an essential insight that we simply have to grasp if we're to see things – and offer care – in deeper ways.

Conclusion

In a health care context, two things really matter:

Firstly, that you are aware that you – and anyone else – chooses which view of the world they want at a particular time – everything depends on how you look at it. You can see cells under a microscope if that is required to solve a problem – but you need always to remember that this is just one view of an incredibly complex reality.

And secondly, that as a health worker you can choose to see the world in ways you think may be most productive in any given circumstance and consciously work out what the patient's current view is, rather than assume your own view is correct.

Here is an apparently simple example from everyday health care, reported to me by a retired nurse (Vanessa Peutherer, Values Exchange Learning Facilitator) who is intuitively aware of every item in the Toolkit. I offer it here, with step-by-step reference to each part of the Toolkit, as a support for those who prefer to see the method and workings spelt out:

A WORKED EXAMPLE: HOW TO APPLY THE TOOLKIT IN EVERYDAY HEALTH CARE – THE CASE OF THE TED STOCKINGS

'I took care of a lady (let's call her Judy) who was labelled as "difficult" because she was seen as "non-compliant" with hospital policy. Judy had chosen not to wear her anti-embolism stockings (thromboembolism-deterrent hose or TED stockings) post-operatively. Others started to avoid this lady during the shift. Having taken the time to speak to her intently and involve her in her choices in an informed way, I was able to realise that she was not informed of the risks versus benefit, and that she found the stockings itchy and painful (because, it emerged, she was wearing the wrong size stocking). After surgery to her knee, her leg had swelled and she just needed a larger stocking. I told her that it was completely her choice as to whether she wore them or not, and that she was free to remove them whenever she wanted to, this was totally up to her, and I respected her choices.

After listening to her I asked her whether she would like me to apply some moisturiser and measure her for a different pair. She agreed and decided eventually that she wanted to wear them. No one had bothered to ask her why she took them off. By giving her informed choice, showing compassion and giving her the opportunity to talk about her feelings we managed to solve the problem in equal partnership.'

Vanessa also told me that she purposely chose to take tea with Judy, spending about 15 minutes with her, giving her full attention. While she was doing this she was aware of other staff walking past, obviously disapproving of what she was doing.

Let's take the Toolkit items one by one:

TOOLKIT ITEM ONE: PRACTICE MINDFUL LABELLING

Vanessa was well-aware that Judy was labelled as 'difficult', and because she was aware, she knew there was more to Judy, and the reasons for her behaviour, than simple 'non-compliance'.

'Difficult' is rather obviously a label, because it is negative. But it's important to remember that every description of another person is a label, even the most positive and even if we wholeheartedly agree with the label.

Mindful labelling is a caution: there is always much more underneath the label, and if we want to offer creative care – in fact if we want to be fair to other people – we should continually be aware of this.

TOOLKIT ITEM TWO: ALWAYS TRY TO UNDERSTAND YOUR OWN AND OTHER PEOPLE'S DECISION BUBBLES

This is so very important. Vanessa took the trouble to think about the causes of Judy's 'non-compliance': was she really being stroppy and pig-headed, or was there more to Judy's decision making than met the eye? Of course, the latter was true, it always is.

Judy had created a decision bubble: 'I don't want to wear the TED stockings.' As we know, decision bubbles do not spring out of thin air, they are formed from complex forces, most beyond our consciousness. For Judy, there was lack of information, a sense of frustration, a sense of neglect, a lack of control, physical pain and no real acknowledgement that she was valued by the other health carers.

To her great credit, Vanessa took the trouble to look outside Judy's decision bubble, to comprehend its causes. And because she did she was able to empathise, to see her as a complex and sensitive being, and to understand exactly why her decision bubble made sense to Judy. Vanessa did not jump to conclusions, rather she looked at the evidence, could see what the problems were, could see what informed Judy's decision and as a consequence could connect with Judy and offer her health promoting choices.

TOOLKIT ITEM THREE: UNDERSTAND THAT WORK FOR HEALTH IS WORK TO CREATE AUTONOMY

This is a perfect example of focussing on autonomy in health care. Not only does it empower both the patient and the carer, it makes the clinical intervention easier and more effective as well.

Why wouldn't you try to create autonomy as your first focus?

This is not to say that 'create autonomy' is the answer to everything – life is much more complicated than this and, where it is, you need rich, connected frameworks to help you work things through. If, for example, Judy's partner were

(Continued)

(Continued)

for some reason against the stockings, creating Judy's autonomy without looking at the partner's decision bubble, is not a complete answer, and may even make things worse. Nonetheless, 'create autonomy' should always be the starting point for thoughtful health care.

TOOLKIT ITEM FOUR: USE CONNECTED FRAMEWORKS TO GUIDE YOUR THOUGHT AND PRACTICE

This is a good example of how to use the Foundations Template discussed in Chapter 5.

You may recall that the Foundations Template uses an image of a stage made up out of five boxes, each of which can be specified in practical detail, with the aim of making more of the patient's life-enhancing potentials a reality. Instinctively, without using the template as a checklist, Vanessa asked: what are Judy's basic needs? (Choice. Respect. Comfort. Safety.) What information does Judy need? (To know risks and benefits. To know that she has the option of a different pair of stockings.) What education would benefit Judy? (To understand the clinical rationale properly.) What sense of belonging does Judy need? (Not to feel that she is a problem to the other health carers. To feel that she is the same person she is outside the hospital.) And finally, what are her special needs? What clinical intervention(s) might she most benefit from? (Properly fitting, effective stockings, that do not irritate her.)

TOOLKIT ITEM FIVE: WORK OUT WHAT YOU ARE COMMITTED TO AND ACT ON IT

This is a continuing process – it shouldn't be taken as a given. In Judy's case there was no need for Vanessa to reassess her commitment to working intelligently for health, but she must always be open to the possibility that her commitment might change, and that it might be right that it does.

TOOLKIT ITEM SIX: REMEMBER THAT CULTURE CHANGE IS POSSIBLE

It is very hard to imagine deep cultural change in health systems, for the many reasons explained in this book. But nothing lasts forever. Everything changes. And the only way we can influence the process is to stand up for what we believe in, even if it will cost us personally. Vanessa knew her colleagues did not approve of her approach, but she had faith, resolve and courage.

She certainly influenced Judy for the better. Possibly, by setting a thoughtful, caring example that actually worked, she influenced her colleagues too.

TOOLKIT ITEM SEVEN: REMEMBER THAT IT IS UP TO YOU WHETHER YOU SEE THINGS AS SEPARATE OR CONNECTED

This is so important too. Judy could have been seen as an 'embolism risk', and nothing else. Possibly she was seen this way by some. There are health carers who find it easiest to think in this reductive style. That is their choice, and their loss. Other health workers, like Vanessa, can choose to try to appreciate the intricate wiring of life, aware that it will always only be a part of the story, but will be glad they made the effort, and so much richer for gaining a deeper view of the world around them.

Thoughtful, kind health workers see the meadow, not the goblin.

SUMMARY OF CHAPTER 8 – THE TOOLKIT

TOOLKIT ITEM ONE: PRACTICE MINDFUL LABELLING

TOOLKIT ITEM TWO: ALWAYS TRY TO UNDERSTAND YOUR OWN AND OTHER PEOPLE'S DECISION BUBBLES

TOOLKIT ITEM THREE: UNDERSTAND THAT WORK FOR HEALTH IS WORK TO CREATE AUTONOMY

TOOLKIT ITEM FOUR: USE CONNECTED FRAMEWORKS TO GUIDE YOUR THOUGHT AND PRACTICE

TOOLKIT ITEM FIVE: WORK OUT WHAT YOU ARE COMMITTED TO AND ACT ON IT

TOOLKIT ITEM SIX: REMEMBER THAT CULTURE CHANGE IS POSSIBLE

TOOLKIT ITEM SEVEN: REMEMBER THAT IT IS UP TO YOU WHETHER YOU SEE THINGS AS SEPARATE OR CONNECTED

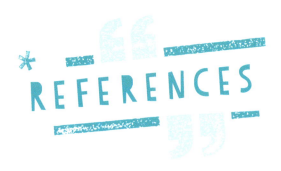

REFERENCES

1. Seedhouse, D.F. (2005) *Values-based Decision-making for the Caring Professions*. Chichester: Wiley.
2. Seedhouse, D.F. (2001) *Health: The Foundations for Achievement*, 2nd edn. Chichester: Wiley.
3. Seedhouse, D.F. (2009) *Ethics: The Heart of Health Care*, 3rd edn. Chichester: Wiley.
4. Seedhouse, D.F. (2003) *Health Promotion: Philosophy, Prejudice and Practice*, 2nd edn. Chichester: Wiley.
5. Seedhouse, D.F. (1994) *Fortress NHS: A Philosophical Review of the National Health Service*. Chichester: Wiley.
6. NHS (2015) *Principles and Values that Guide the NHS*. Available at: www.nhs.uk/NHSEngland/thenhs/about/Pages/nhscoreprinciples.aspx (accessed 10 June 2016).
7. MS Society (2014) *Sativex Likely to be Available in Wales, but not England*. Available at: www.mssociety.org.uk/ms-news/2014/08/sativex-likely-be-available-wales-not-england (accessed 6 October 2016).
8. *The Guardian* (2014) *Cannabis Drug for Multiple Sclerosis 'Too Costly' for England but not Wales*. Available at: www.theguardian.com/society/2014/oct/08/drug-multiple-sclerosis-england-wales-nice (accessed 6 October 2016).
9. *The Telegraph* (2012) *NHS Facing £15.7bn for Rising Number of Clinical Negligence Claims*. Available at: www.telegraph.co.uk/news/politics/9065534/NHS-facing-15.7bn-for-rising-number-of-clinical-negligence-claims.html (accessed 6 October 2016).
10. NHS (2015) *NHS Litigation Authority: Report and Accounts 2014/2015*. Available at: www.nhsla.com/aboutus/Documents/NHS%20LA%20Annual%20Report%20and%20Accounts%202014-15.pdf (accessed 6 October 2016).
11. Fann, W. (2014) *Tardive Dyskinesia: Research & Treatment*. New York: Springer.

12. Breggin, P. (1993) *Toxic Psychiatry. Drugs and Electroconvulsive Therapy: The Truth and the Better* Alternatives. London: Harper Collins.
13. Mansharamani, V. (01/06/2016) *Superbugs: The $100 Trillion Risk*. Available at: http://fortune.com/2016/06/01/antibiotic-superbugs-bacteria-e-coli/ (accessed 6 October 2016).
14. *Express* (2016) *Warning: Rise of SUPERBUGS Resistant to Antibiotics Poses 'Bigger Risk than CANCER'*. Available at: www.express.co.uk/life-style/health/671748/rise-of-superbugs-resistant-antibiotics-bigger-risk-cancer (accessed 6 October 2016).
15. Bentall, R.P. (2010) *Doctoring the Mind: Why Psychiatric Treatments Fail*. London: Penguin.
16. Action Against Medical Accidents (n.d.) *Case Studies*. Available at: www.avma.org.uk/patient-stories/case-studies/ (accessed 6 October 2016).
17. South Essex Partnership University NHS Foundation Trust (SEPT) (n.d.) *NHS Core Values*. Available at: www.sept.nhs.uk/about-us/nhs-constitution/nhs-core-values/ (accessed 6 October 2016).
18. NHS Institute for Innovation and Improvement (2013) *The Policy Framework*. Available at: http://webarchive.nationalarchives.gov.uk/20150401212609/http://www.institute.nhs.uk/patient_experience/guide/the_policy_framework.html (accessed 6 October 2016).
19. Greater Manchester West NHS (n.d.) *Our Vision, Values and Objectives*. Available at: www.gmw.nhs.uk/our-values (accessed 6 October 2016).
20. NHS England (2012) *Compassion in Practice: Our Culture of Compassionate Care*. Available at: www.england.nhs.uk/nursingvision/compassion/ (accessed 6 October 2016).
21. Department of Health and NHS Commissioning Board (2012) *Compassion in Practice. Nursing, Midwifery and Care Staff: Our Vision and Strategy*. Available at: www.england.nhs.uk/wp-content/uploads/2012/12/compassion-in-practice.pdf (accessed 6 October 2016).
22. Roach, M. S. (1984) *Caring: The Human Mode of Being, Implications for Nursing*. Ottawa: The Canadian Hospital Association Press.
23. Bradshaw, A. (2015) 'An analysis of England's nursing policy on compassion and the 6Cs: the hidden presence of M. Simone Roach's model of caring', *Nursing Inquiry*, 23 (1): 78–85. Available at: http://onlinelibrary.wiley.com/doi/10.1111/nin.12107/full (accessed 6 October 2016).
24. Nursing: A World of Caring [blog] (n.d.) *S. Roach*. Available at: https://jaimesorianorn.wordpress.com/lecture-handouts (accessed 6 October 2016).
25. Francis, R. (2013) *The Report of the Mid Staffordshire NHS Foundation Trust Public Inquiry*. London: The Stationery Office. Available at: http://webarchive.nationalarchives.gov.uk/20150407084003/http://www.midstaffspublicinquiry.com/report (accessed 11 October 2016).

26. Keough, B. (2013) *Review into the Quality of Care and Treatment Provided by 14 Hospital Trusts in England: Overview Report.* Available at: www.nhs.uk/NHSEngland/bruce-keogh-review/Documents/outcomes/keogh-review-final-report.pdf (accessed 11 October 2016).
27. Berwick, D. (2013) *A Promise to Learn – A Commitment to Act. Improving the Safety of Patients in England.* Available at: www.gov.uk/government/uploads/system/uploads/attachment_data/file/226703/Berwick_Report.pdf (accessed 11 October 2016).
28. The Telegraph (2013) *Mid Staffordshire Trust inquiry: How the Care Scandal Unfolded.* Available at: www.telegraph.co.uk/news/health/news/9851763/Mid-Staffordshire-Trust-inquiry-how-the-care-scandal-unfolded.html (accessed 6 October 2016).
29. The British Psychological Society and Division of Occupational Psychology (2014) *Implementing culture change within the NHS: Contributions from Occupational Psychology.* Available at: www.bps.org.uk/system/files/userfiles/Division%20of%20Occupational%20Psychology/public/17689_cat-1658.pdf (accessed 6 October 2016).
30. HR Magazine (2015) *Can Recruiting Values Go Too Far?* Available at: www.hrmagazine.co.uk/article-details/can-recruiting-for-values-go-too-far (accessed 13 June 2016).
31. Skills for Health (2015) *Is Values Based Recruitment Wasted Time and Money?* Available at: www.skillsforhealth.org.uk/news/blog/item/258-is-values-based-recruitment-wasted-time-and-money (accessed 13 June 2016).
32. Health Education England (2014) *Values Based Recruitment.* Available at: http://hee.nhs.uk/work-programmes/values-based-recruitment/ (accessed 6 October 2016).
33. Goode, J. (2014) *Value Based Recruitment Toolkit.* Available at www.skillsforcare.org.uk/Document-library/Finding-and-keeping-workers/Practical-toolkits/Values-based-recruitment/Final-report.pdf (accessed 26 April 2017).
34. *Why We Think it's OK to Cheat and Steal (Sometimes)* (2009). Available at: www.youtube.com/watch?v=nUdsTizSxSI (accessed 6 October 2016).
35. NHS Employers (cited in a presentation by: Lydia Larcum, Senior HR Lead – Staff Engagement & Health and Wellbeing, York Teaching Hospital NHS Foundation Trust. Lydia.Larcum@nhsemployers.org).
36. Coca-Cola Company (n.d.) *Mission, Vision & Values.* Available at: www.coca-colacompany.com/our-company/mission-vision-values (accessed 6 October 2016).
37. Coca-Cola Company (2007) *Coca-Cola: Drinking the World Dry.* Available at: www.waronwant.org/news/campaigns-news/15153-coca-cola-drinking-the-world-dry (accessed 6 October 2016).
38. The Telegraph (2015) *Man Boils Coca Cola to Show How Much Sugar is in One Bottle.* Available at: www.telegraph.co.uk/foodanddrink/11447515/

Man-boils-Coca-Cola-to-show-how-much-sugar-is-in-one-bottle.html (accessed 6 October 2016).

39. Forbes (2016) *The Just 100: America's Best Corporate Citizens*. Available at: www.forbes.com/just-companies/#669f0a8d9ab9 (accessed 19 January 2017).

40. Mission Statement of McDonalds. Available at: www.strategicmanagementinsight.com/mission-statements/mcdonalds-mission-statement.html (accessed 17 January 2017).
McDonalds (n.d.) Our Ambition. Available at: www.aboutmcdonalds.com/content/mcd/our_company/our-ambition.html (accessed 6 October 2016).

41. *Why McDonald's is McF*cked: Weapons of Mass Distraction* (2015). Available at: www.youtube.com/watch?v=B3swf0Sj5bc (accessed 12 October 2016).

42. Army (n.d.) *Join as an Officer*. Available at: www.army.mod.uk/infantry/regiments/parachute/24346.aspx (accessed 6 October 2016).

43. History Channel (n.d.) *Battle of Gallipoli*. Available at: www.history.com/topics/world-war-i/battle-of-gallipoli (accessed 6 October 2016).

44. Lavender Primary School (n.d.) *Vision and Values*. Available at: www.lavender.enfield.sch.uk/page/?pid=35 (accessed 6 October 2016).

45. Oliver, D. (2016) 'Values statements aren't worth the paper', *BMJ*, 353: i3103. Available at: www.bmj.com/content/353/bmj.i3103 (accessed 6 October 2016).

46. NHS Employers (n.d.) Available at: www.nhsemployers.org/your-workforce/recruit/employer-led-recruitment/values-based-recruitment (accessed 6 October 2016).

47. University of Birmingham (n.d.) *Values Based Recruitment: What Works, for Whom, Why and in What Way?* Available at: www.birmingham.ac.uk/schools/social-policy/departments/health-services-management-centre/research/projects/2015/values-based-recruitment.aspx (accessed 12 October 2016).

48. Jones, H. (2104) 'Putting the 6Cs at the heart of nurse education', *Nursing Times*, 110 (37): 12–14.

49. Health Education England (2013) *Values Based Recruitment Programme Equality Analysis*. Available at: www.hee.nhs.uk/sites/default/files/documents/HEE_National_VBR_EandD.pdf (accessed 19 January 2017).

50. *The Guardian* (2016) There's a long list of NHS inquiries, but what have they actually changed? Available at: www.theguardian.com/healthcare-network/2016/mar/04/national-health-service-nhs-inquiries-what-have-they-changed (accessed 6 October 2016).

51. Cost of Living (2016) *Is the NHS Really Suffering a Crisis of Compassion?* Available at: www.cost-ofliving.net/is-the-nhs-really-suffering-a-crisis-of-compassion (accessed 6 October 2016).

52. Wagner A. Kamakura, Jose A. Mazzon. (1991) 'Value segmentation: a model for the measurement of values and value systems', *Journal of Consumer Research*, 18 (2): 208–218.

53. United Nations University (2012) *Residual Colonialism in the 21st Century.* Available at: http://unu.edu/publications/articles/residual-colonialism-in-the-21st-century.html (accessed 6 October 2016).
54. Hough, R. (2003) *Captain James Cook: A Biography.* New York: W.W. Norton.
55. Izzard, E. (2006) *Do You Have a Flag?* Available at: www.youtube.com/watch?v=UTduy7Qkvk8 (12 October 2016).
56. Althusser, L. (2008) *On Ideology.* London: Verso.
57. Cassirer, E. (1956) *An Essay on Man.* New York: Doubleday Anchor, p. 43.
58. *One Flew Over The Cuckoo's Nest: Doctor Fishing Scene.* Available at: www.youtube.com/watch?v=QH4NRIDjRjk (accessed 19 January 2017).
59. Goffman, E. (1961) *Asylums.* New York: Doubleday.
60. Hilgard, E.R., Atkinson, R.L. and Atkinson, R.C. (1979) *Introduction to Psychology*, 7th edn. New York: Harcourt Brace Jovanovich.
61. The Guardian (2009) *When Smoking was Cool, Cheap, Legal and Socially Acceptable.* Available at: www.theguardian.com/lifeandstyle/2009/apr/01/tobacco-industry-marketing (accessed 12 October 2016).
62. Smil, V. *(2013) Should We Eat Meat? Evolution and Consequences of Modern Carnivory.* Oxford*: Wiley-Blackwell.*
63. *Bayer, R. (1987) Homosexuality and American Psychiatry: The Politics of Diagnosis.* Princeton: Princeton University Press.
64. Nightingale, F. (1898) 'Ventilation and warming', in *Notes on Nursing: What it is, and what it is not.* Available at: www.nursingplanet.com/nightingale/ventilatin_and_warming.html (accessed 7 October 2016).
65. *Deadline News* (2012) *Scots Hospital Windows Locked Shut to Stop Patients Falling Out.* Available at: www.deadlinenews.co.uk/2012/03/16/scots-hospital-windows-locked-shut-to-stop-patients-falling-out (accessed 7 October 2016).
66. Nightingale, F. (1898) 'Variety', in *Notes on Nursing: What it is, and what it is not.* Available at: www.nursingplanet.com/nightingale/variety.html (accessed 7 October 2016).
67. Moby (1999) *Play.* Mute Records. (sleeve notes).
68. James Burke, *Connections.* Available at: https://en.wikipedia.org/wiki/Connections_(TV_series) (accessed 26 April 2017).
69. Russell, B. (2007) *The Problems of Philosophy.* New Jersey: Cosimo Classics.
70. Institute of Chronic Pain (n.d.) *Understanding Chronic Pain.* Available at: www.instituteforchronicpain.org/understanding-chronic-pain/what-is-chronic-pain (accessed 26 April 2017).
    Health Central (n.d.) *Hyperalgesia: It Hurts Everywhere!* Available at: www.healthcentral.com/chronic-pain/c/240381/159492/hyperalgesia-hurts (accessed 12 October 2016).
71. Emanuelson, J. (n.d.) *The Needle Pain Page.* Available at: www.needlephobia.com/ (accessed 12 October 2016).

72. Gloucestershire Hospitals NHS Foundation Trust (n.d.) *How do Different Aspects of the Ward Influence the Patient?* Available at: www.gloucestershireacademy.nhs.uk/bristol_st/docs/How%20do%20different%20aspects%20of%20the%20ward%20influence%20the%20patient.pdf (accessed 12 October 2016).
73. *Daily Mail* (2014) *Flowers Ban at 9 in 10 Hospitals: Increasing Numbers Introduce Rules after Concerns Blooms Spread Germs and Create Extra Work for Nurses.* Available at: www.dailymail.co.uk/news/article-2591250/Flowers-ban-9-10-hospitals-concerns-blooms-spread-germs.html#ixzz3vuMnFYmT (accessed 12 October 2016).
74. Science Daily (2009) *Should Flowers be Banned in Hospitals?* 17 December. Available at: www.sciencedaily.com/releases/2009/12/091216203449.htm (accessed 12 October 2016).
75. Lorenz, E.N. *(1963)* 'The predictability of hydrodynamic flow', *Transactions of the New York Academy of Sciences,* 25 (4): 409–32.
76. Buchanan, A. (2011) *Better than Human.* Oxford: Oxford University Press.
77. Power, M. (2004) *The Risk Management of Everything: Rethinking the politics of uncertainty.* London: Demos.
78. Imlach Gunasekara, F.H. (2010) 'Patients should be able to choose who sits on their beds', *British Medical Journal*, 340: doi 10.1136/bmj.c1495. Available at: www.bmj.com/rapid-responses?sort_by=field_highwire_a_epubdate_value_1&sort_order=ASC&items_per_page=5&page=15498 (accessed 19 January 2017).
79. Illich, I. (1995) *Deschooling Society.* London: Marion Boyars Publishers Ltd.
80. *Israeli Activists: Reject Mandatory Military Service: Interview with Amit Gilutzle* Available at: www.youtube.com/watch?v=CbNsVGUti9c (accessed 13 October 2016).
81. Sir Ken Robinson (2007) *Do Schools Kill Creativity?* TED Talks. Available at: www.youtube.com/watch?v=iG9CE55wbtY (accessed 13 August 2014).
82. Sir Ken Robinson (n.d.) *How Schools Kill Creativity.* Available at: https://creativesystemsthinking.wordpress.com/2015/04/26/ken-robinson-how-schools-kill-creativity (accessed 13 October 2016).
83. *Suli Breaks – Why I Hate School But Love Education.* Available at: www.youtube.com/watch?v=y_ZmM7zPLyI (accessed 13 October 2016).
84. *The Independent* (2015) *Finland schools: Subjects Scrapped and Replaced with 'Topics' as Country Reforms its Education System.* Available at: www.independent.co.uk/news/world/europe/finland-schools-subjects-are-out-and-topics-are-in-as-country-reforms-its-education-system-10123911.html (accessed 13 October 2016).
85. *The Telegraph* (2010) *Frano Selak: 'World's Luckiest Man' Gives Away His Lottery Fortune.* Available at: www.telegraph.co.uk/news/newstopics/how

aboutthat/7721985/Frano-Selak-worlds-luckiest-man-gives-away-his-lottery-fortune.html (accessed 13 October 2016).

86. Listverse (2013) *9 Unluckiest People Ever.* Available at: http://listverse.com/2013/01/05/10-unluckiest-people-ever/ (accessed 13 October 2016).

87. *The Independent* (2015) *Nagasaki Anniversary: Tsutomu Yamaguchi, the Man Who Survived both Hiroshima and Nagasaki.* Available at: www.independent.co.uk/news/world/asia/nagasaki-anniversary-meet-tsutomu-yamaguchi-the-man-who-survived-both-hiroshima-and-nagasaki-10447342.html (accessed 13 October 2016).

88. *The Telegraph* (2014) *Please don't call me 'Inspiring' just because I have a disability.* Available at: www.telegraph.co.uk/men/thinking-man/11261231/Please-dont-call-me-inspiring-just-because-I-have-a-disability.html (accessed 13 October 2016).

89. Keller, H. (1905) *The Story of My Life.* New York: Doubleday, Page & Company. p. 11. Available at: http://digital.library.upenn.edu/women/keller/life/life.html (accessed 15 March 2016).

90. Shakespeare, W. *The Tragedy of Hamlet Prince of Denmark. The Harvard Classics.* 1909–14. Act II, Scene II. Available at: www.bartleby.com/46/2 (accessed 26 April 2017).

91. *The Guardian* (2014) *The Case Against Human Rights.* Available at: www.theguardian.com/news/2014/dec/04/-sp-case-against-human-rights (accessed 13 October 2016).

92. Smith, G. (2012) *Jeremy Bentham's Attack on Human Rights.* Available at: www.libertarianism.org/publications/essays/excursions/jeremy-benthams-attack-natural-rights (accessed 13 October 2016).

93. *Aboriginal Culture – Politics & Media – Northern Territory Emergency Response (NTER) – 'The Intervention'.* Available at: www.CreativeSpirits.info (accessed 9 October 2016).

94. Dobelli, R. (2010) *Avoid News: Towards a Healthy Diet.* Available at: http://dobelli.com/wp-content/uploads/2010/08/Avoid_News_Part1_TEXT.pdf (accessed 13 October 2016).

95. Postman, N. (2005) *Amusing Ourselves to Death: Public Discourse in the Age of Show Business*. New York: Penguin.

96. Kudaibergenova, T. (2013) 'Developing a Culturally Sensitive Research Ethics in Kyrgyzstan: Culturally Sensitive Method for Obtaining Truly Informed Consent', MS thesis, Union Graduate College (now Clarkson University).

97. Sagan, K. (1997) *Billions and Billions.* New York and Toronto: Ballentine Publishing Group.

98. Sale, K. (n.d.) *Five Facets of a Myth.* Available at: www.primitivism.com/facets-myth.htm (accessed 19 January 2017).

99. Harari, Y.N. (2011) *Sapiens: A Brief History of Humankind*. London: Harvill Secker.
100. Tompkins, P. and Bird, C. (1989) *The Secret Life of Plants*. London: Harper Perennial.
101. Sheldrake, R. and Smart, P. (2000) 'A dog that seems to know when his owner is coming home: videotaped experiments and observations', *Journal of Scientific Exploration*, 14: 233–55.
102. *New York Times* (2016) *Lacking Brains, Plants Can Still Make Good Judgments About Risks*. Available at: www.nytimes.com/2016/07/01/science/pea-plants-risk-assessment.html?_r=0 (accessed 13 October 2016).
103. Hughes, P. and Ferrett, E. (2005) *Introduction to Health and Safety at Work: The Handbook for Students on NEBOSH and Other Introductory H and S Courses*. London: Routledge.
104. Agger, B. (1998) *Critical Social Theories: An Introduction*. Boulder CO: Westview.
105. Stutchbury, K. and Fox, A. (2009) 'Ethics in educational research: introducing a methodological tool for effective ethical analysis', *Cambridge Journal of Education*, 39 (4): 489–504.
106. *The drop-out club for doctors: Why medics are leaving the NHS*. Available at: https://nhsreality.wordpress.com/2014/06/02/the-drop-out-club-for-doctors-why-medics-are-leaving-the-nhs (accessed 13 October 2016).
107. *Daily Mail* (2016) *Missing Junior Doctor 'Left Suicide Note Mentioning Jeremy Hunt' After Walking Out of Hospital Halfway Through Her Shift*. Available at: www.dailymail.co.uk/news/article-3449031/Hopes-fade-missing-junior-doctor-walked-hospital.html (accessed 13 October 2016).
108. Narasimhan, J. (2006) 'Vegan? Sorry, We Have Porcine Heparin on the Menu!', *Anesthesia & Analgesia*, 102 (3): 976.
109. Proctor, R. and Thomsen, L. (2013) *Veganissimo A to Z: A Comprehensive Guide to Identifying and Avoiding Ingredients of Animal Origin in Everyday Products*. New York: The Experiment.
110. NPR (2013) *Is Your Medicine Vegan? Probably Not*. Available at: www.npr.org/sections/health-shots/2013/03/13/174205188/is-your-medicine-vegan-probably-not (accessed 13 October 2016).
111. Strickland, S.R. (2014) 'Suitability of common drugs for patients who avoid animal products', *British Medical Journal*, 348: g401. Available at: www.bmj.com/content/348/bmj.g401/rr/689984 (accessed 13 October 2016).
112. Seedhouse, D. (1991) 'Against medical ethics: a philosopher's view', *Medical Education*, 25 (4): 280–82. Available at: http://onlinelibrary.wiley.com/doi/10.1111/j.1365-2923.1991.tb00066.x/abstract (accessed 13 October 2016).

113. Beauchamp, T. and Childress, J. (2012) *Principles of Biomedical Ethics*, 7th edn. Oxford: Oxford University Press.
114. Clouser, K. and Gert, B. (1990) 'A critique of principlism', *The Journal of Medicine and Philosophy*, 15 (2): 219–36.
115. Bacon, F. (2008) *Francis Bacon: The Major Works* (ed. B. Vickers). Oxford: Oxford World's Classics.
116. Cherry, K. (2016) *The Muller-Lyer Illusion (How it Works)*. Available at: http://psychology.about.com/od/sensationandperception/ss/muller-lyer-illusion.htm (accessed 13 October 2016).
117. Vanderbilt, T. (2014) *How Your Brain Decides Without You.* Available at: http://nautil.us/issue/19/illusions/how-your-brain-decides-without-you (accessed 13 October 2016).
118. American Psychiatric Association. *Diagnostic and Statistical Manual of Mental Disorders (DSM-5).* Available at: www.dsm5.org/psychiatrists/practice/dsm (accessed 19 January 2017).
119. Wishart, I. (2009) *AIR CON: The Seriously Inconvenient Truth About Global Warming.* Available at: www.youtube.com/watch?v=90otAJORkK8 (accessed 13 October 2016).
120. Hobson, K. (2013) 'What sceptics believe': the effects of information and deliberation on climate change scepticism, *Public Understanding of Science*, 22 (4): 1–17.
121. *The Great Global Warming Swindle*. Available at: www.youtube.com/watch?v=D-m09lKtYT4 (accessed 13 October 2016).
122. Orwell, G. (2013) *1984*. London: Penguin.
123. Pet Food Manufacturers' Association (n.d.) *Pet Population 2014*. Available at: www.pfma.org.uk/pet-population-2014 (accessed 19 January 2017).
124. PETA, *Glass Walls*. Available at: www.peta.org/videos/glass-walls-2/ (accessed 13 October 2016).
125. BBC Earth (2014) *Smart Pigs vs Kids – Extraordinary Animals – Series 2 – Earth*. Available at: www.youtube.com/watch?v=mza1EQ6aLdg (accessed 13 October 2016).
126. *The Guardian* (2015) *Industrial Farming is One of the Worst Crimes in History*. Available at: www.theguardian.com/books/2015/sep/25/industrial-farming-one-worst-crimes-history-ethical-question? (accessed 13 October 2016).
127. Campbell, J. (1989) *The Improbable Machine: What the Upheavals in Artificial Intelligence Research Reveal About How the Mind Really Works:* London: Simon and Schuster.
128. Joy, M. (2015) *Toward Rational, Authentic Food Choices (TEDx München).* Available at: www.youtube.com/watch?v=o0VrZPBskpg (accessed 19 January 2017).

129. The Laughing Cow. Available at: www.thelaughingcow.co.uk (accessed 14 October 2016).
130. The Happy Egg Co. Available at: https://thehappyegg.co.uk (accessed 14 October 2016).
131. Humane Slaughter Association (2005) *Gas Killings of Chickens and Turkeys*. Available at: www.hsa.org.uk/downloads/technical-notes/TN12-gas-killing-of-chickens-and-turkeys.pdf (accessed 14 October 2016).
132. *Kristallnacht: Background & Overview*. Available at: www.jewishvirtuallibrary.org/jsource/Holocaust/kristallnacht.html (accessed 14 October 2016).
133. Shah, A. (2011) 'Today, around 21,000 children died around the world', *Global Issues*. Available at: www.globalissues.org/article/715/today-21000-children-died-around-the-world (accessed 19 January 2017).
134. *The Bystander Effect*. Available at: www.youtube.com/watch?v=OSsPfbup0ac (accessed 19 January 2017).
135. Ethical Consumer (2016) *Tax Avoidance Rankings*. Available at: www.ethical-consumer.org/ethicalcampaigns/taxjusticecampaign/taxavoidancerankings.aspx (accessed 19 January 2017).
136. *The Iraq Inquiry*. Available at: www.iraqinquiry.org.uk/the-report (accessed 19 January 2017).
137. Big Think, *How Too Much Education Can Result in Ignorance*. Available at: http://bigthink.com/praxis/youre-more-ignorant-than-you-think-you-are (accessed 14 October 2016).
138. *What are Some of the Best Examples of Beliefs That Were Once Thought to Be True But Are Now Known to be Completely Wrong?* Available at: www.quora.com/What-are-some-of-the-best-examples-of-beliefs-that-were-once-thought-to-be-true-but-are-now-known-to-be-completely-wrong (accessed 14 October 2016).
139. Ariely, D. (2009) *Why We Think it's OK to Cheat and Steal (Sometimes)*. Available at: www.youtube.com/watch?v=nUdsTizSxSI (accessed 14 October 2016).
140. Stevens, L., *Does Mental Illness Exist?* Available at: www.antipsychiatry.org/exist.htm) (accessed 14 October 2016).
141. ScienceBlogs (2013) *Most Scientific Theories are Wrong*. Available at: http://scienceblogs.com/startswithabang/2013/05/31/most-scientific-theories-are-wrong (accessed 14 October 2016).
142. Nemade, R., Staats Reiss, N. and Dombeck, M. (2007) *Sociology of Depression: Effects of Culture*. Available at: www.mentalhelp.net/articles/sociology-of-depression-effects-of-culture (accessed 14 October 2016).
143. Dawkins, R. (January–February 1997) *Is Science a Religion?* American Humanist Association. Available at: www.2think.org/Richard_Dawkins_Is_Science_A_Religion.shtml (accessed 15 March 2008).

144. *Is it Really True that No Two Snowflakes are Alike?* Available at: www.its.caltech.edu/~atomic/snowcrystals/alike/alike.htm (accessed 14 October 2016).

145. Popper, K. (2002) *Conjectures and Refutations: The Growth of Scientific Knowledge.* New York and London: Routledge.

146. *What is Mindfulness and How Will it Help Me?* Available at: http://bemindful.co.uk (accessed 14 October 2016).

147. *6 Mindfulness Exercises You Can Try Today.* Available at: www.pocket-mindfulness.com/6-mindfulness-exercises-you-can-try-today (accessed 14 October 2016).

148. Aldersey-Williams, H. (2016) *Tide: The Science and Lore of the Greatest Force on Earth.* London: Penguin.

149. Hainer, R. (2010) *Social Smokers aren't Hooked on Nicotine, Just Smoking.* Available at: http://edition.cnn.com/2010/HEALTH/04/24/social.smokers (accessed 14 October 2016).

150. Seedhouse, D.F. (2005) *Values-based Decision-making for the Caring Professions.* Chichester: Wiley.

151. Ament, A. (2010) 'Beyond Vibrations: The Deaf Experience in Music.' *Gapers Block.* Available at: http://gapersblock.com/transmission/2010/07/22/beyond_vibrations_the_deaf_musical_experience (accessed 14 October 2016).

152. Gibbs, G. (1988) *Learning by Doing: A Guide to Teaching and Learning Methods.* London: FEU.

153. Mannion, R. and Davies, H.T. (2015) 'Cultures of silence and cultures of voice: the role of whistleblowing in healthcare organisations', *International Journal of Health Policy and Management*, 4 (8): 503–5.

154. Basford, L. and Slevin, O. (2003) *Theory and Practice of Nursing: An Integrated Approach to Caring Practice*, 2nd Edition (Campion Integrated Studies). Andover, Hampshire: Cengage.

155. NHS England (2015) *How Much Do Clinicians Support Patient Activations? A Survey of Clinician Attitudes and Behaviours Towards People Taking an Active Role in their Health and Care.* Available at: www.england.nhs.uk/wp-content/uploads/2015/11/cspam-report.pdf (accessed 14 October 2016).

156. Nesta (2012) *Working Towards People Powered Health: Insights from Practitioners.* Available at: www.nesta.org.uk/sites/default/files/working_for_co-production_in_healthcare.pdf (accessed 14 October 2016).

157. Community Living (2016) *Risk-averse staff are undermining the aims of the Mental Capacity Act.* Available at: www.cl-initiatives.co.uk/risk-averse-staff-undermining-aims-mental-capacity-act (accessed 14 October 2016).

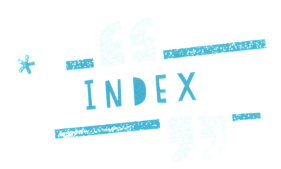

INDEX

4-hour waiting time, 12
6Cs, 7–11, 20, 30, 112
9/11 attacks, 81, 83
1984, 134

A&E (Accident and Emergency), 12
Aboriginal and Torres Strait Island People, 79
access, to services, 6
Accident and Emergency (A&E), 12
accountability, 7
ADHD (attention deficit hyperactivity disorder), 39, 47, 48, 153
advocacy, 172
agency staff, 24
Air Asia Flight QZ 8501, 81
air travel, 26–27
albinism, 77
Aldersley-Williams, Hugh, 150–51
Althusser, Louis, 37–38
Alzheimer's disease, 55, 165–66
Amusing Ourselves to Death, 82
animals, 16, 133, 134–37, 152
anorexia, 4
anti-biotics, 7
anti-coagulants, 110, 116
antipsychotic drugs, 7
appearance, 50–2, 55, 59, 161
Ariely, Dan, 141
Army, 16–17, 31
asthma, 110, 111, 112
attention deficit hyperactivity disorder (ADHD), 9, 47, 48, 153
Australia, 79–80
autonomy, 104, 106, 107, 108, 109, 111, 112, 113, 114, 126, 154, 165–67, 173, 176, 181–83

Backster, Cleve, 97
Bacon, Francis, 129–30
Beauchamp, T., 126, 127–28

Beckham, David, 74
beneficence, 126–27
Bennett, Viv, 8
Bentham, Jeremy, 79
Big Bang, 142
Big Brother, 83
Big Think, 139
bipolar disorder, 61
Bird, Christopher, 96, 98
books, 85
brainwashing, 73
British Army, 16–17, 31
Buchanan, Allen, 68–9
Buddhism, 90–1, 93
Burke, James, 44

Calamity John Lyne, 75
Campbell, Jeremy, 135
capacity, 175–76
carbon dioxide (CO2), 133, 143
care, 8
carers, 3–4
carnism, 135–36
cars, 69
Cassirer, Ernst, 38
Charlie Hebdo, 85
child abuse, 80
children, 138–39
Childress, J., 126, 127–28
climate change, 89, 132, 133, 142
clinical negligence, 6
Clouser, K., 126
CNN, 81, 155
CO2 (carbon dioxide), 133, 143
Coca Cola Company, 14–15
cochineal, 117
cognitive dissonance, 131
cognitive distortion, 138
colonisation, 36–37, 38

colour, 51
commitment, 15, 20, 168–73, 182
communication, 8
compassion, 8, 9–10, 20, 24, 30, 60, 70, 103, 109, 180
Compassion in Practice, 8
competence, 8
compliance, 153, 180, 181
connected frameworks, 167–68, 182
Connections, 44
connectness, 42–5, 47, 49, 146, 162, 171–79, 182
consent, informed, 86
control, 144, 163
Cook, James, 36
co-production, 174
core values, 8
Country Baskets, 66
courage, 8, 10, 17, 20
creativity, 9
cross infection, 70
Crossan, Rob, 77
culture change, 109, 173–78, 182
Cummings, Jane, 7–8
curry, 4–5

Daily Mail, 66–7, 85
Daily Telegraph, 12, 74–75
Dawkins, Richard, 143
Deaf Smith County, 98
deafness, 108, 161
death, 161
decision bubbles, 159–64, 181
delusion
   appearance as, 52
   ethics, 115, 122, 127
   indicators of, 132–45
   luck, 76–7
   nature, 95, 98
   progress, 89, 90, 93
   schools, 71–2
   separateness, 43–4, 103–4, 108, 109, 127
   types of, 129–32
   values, 59–60, 64 *see also* values
dementia, 24, 110, 175
democracy, 18, 25
Department of Health, 66
depression, 4, 70, 143
Diagnostic and Statistical Manual of Mental Disorders (DSM), 133
diagnostic labels, 153–4
dialysis, 110, 127
'difficult' patients, 41, 153, 180, 181
dignity, 8, 22, 23, 26, 103, 111–12
dilemmas, 110–11, 116–17, 128
disability, 77–8, 100, 104
disease, 88, 102, 104, 106–113 *see also* illness

Dobelli, Rolf, 80–2, 85
doctors, 115
dogs, 97
Donne, John, 87–8
doublethink, 134–38
dramatic ethics, 120, 124, 128
drugs, 7, 117
DSM (Diagnostic and Statistical Manual of Mental Disorders), 133
Dunning David, 141
Durkin, Martin, 133

economic rights, 79
education, 117–19
English, 73
environment, 89
equality, 1, 2, 103
ethical grid, 118, 153–54, 168
ethics
   case study, 122–23
   delusion, 115, 121, 124
   dramatic ethics, 120, 124, 128
   ethical dilemmas, 110–11, 115,–16, 127
   ethics committees, 86, 87, 101, 119
   ethics education, 117–19
   four principles fallacy, 126–27, 152
   in the general sense, 120, 121–22, 125
   persisting ethics, 120–21, 124, 128, 153
   personal moral commitment, 172–73
evidence, 13, 21–2, 27, 66, 83, 92, 102, 103, 130, 132–33, 142, 156, 158–59, 170
external conditions, 51

Facebook, 84
families, 3–4
farming, 98, 134–37
Finland, 74
flags, 36–7
flowers, 41, 66–7
Food Safety Act (1990), 5
Ford, Frank, 98
Foundation Status, 12
Foundations Template *see Health: The Foundations for Achievement*
four principles fallacy, 126–27, 152
foxgloves, 148–49
France, Raoul, 96
Francis Report, 8, 11, 12, 24–25, 35, 174, 176
French Revolution, 82

Gallipoli, 17
gay, 33, 41, 48, 142
gelatin, 117
genetics, 88
Gert, B, 126
global warming, 133 *see also* climate change

goals, patient, 169
Gove, Michael, 140
The Great Global Warming Swindle, 133
groups, 87
The Guardian, 79

hailing, 37
Happy Egg Company, 136-37
Harari, Y.N., 94
hard shoulders, 140
Hawkins, Stephen, 78
health, 102-4
Health Education England (HEE), 13, 21
health promotion, 5, 154-58
Health: The Foundations for Achievement, 105, 106, 107
higher education, 20
Hiskey, Syd, 24
homosexuality, 33, 142
honesty, 22, 59, 60
hospitals, 3-4, 54-7, 63, 66-7, 103
Hough, Richard, 36-37
human rights, 2, 78-9
hunter gatherers, 94
Huxley, Aldous, 83

Idols of the Cave, 129-30
Idols of the Marketplace, 129-30
Idols of the Theater, 129-30
Idols of the Tribe, 129-30
ignorance, 141
Illich, Ivan, 72-3
illness, 40-1, 53, 102-4, 105-14, 153, 164 *see also* disease; mental illness
The Impossible Machine, 135
individuality, 86-8, 99
information glut, 83
informed consent, 86
injections, 54
injury, 68, 69, 104, 105, 106, 108, 131, 157, 158
integrity, 14
interpretation, 53, 63, 132, 147, 148, 179
inventions, 44
Israel, 73
Izard, Eddie, 37

Japan, 143
Jews, 138
Joy, Dr Melanie, 135-36, 138
junior doctors, 115
justice, 126-28

Keller, Helen, 78
Kenny, Emma, 66
kidney disease, 110
Kristallnacht, 138

Kudaibergenov, Tamara, 86
Kyrgyzstan, 86, 87

labels, 23, 29, 30, 32-49, 64, 71, 73, 76, 116, 132, 146, 147, 152-54
lactose, 117
Laughing Cow, 136
legislation, 156-58
life expectancy, 88
Listverse.com, 75
Little Ice Age, 44
logic, 134, 159
The Long Chain, 44
Lord, Charles, 141
luck, 74-6
Lyne, John, 75

magazines, 85
Mann, Robert, 227
Maoris, 37
mathematics, 71-3
Mazie, Steven, 139
McCartney, Paul, 137
McDonalds, 15-16, 31
McPherson, Susan, 24
meat, 5, 25-6, 41, 48, 135-36
medicine, 90, 115
Mental Capacity Act 2005, 175
mental illness, 40, 41, 47, 48, 132, 133, 142-43
Mid-Staffordshire scandal, 11-12, 24, 25, 102
military technology, 90
mindful immersion, 150
mindful labelling, 147, 152-8, 181, 183
mindful observation, 149
mindfulness, 148-49
mindless labelling *see* mindful labelling
Moby, 42-43
moon, 150
moral commitment, 172-73
morality *see* ethics
Muller-Lyon Effect, 113(fig)
multiple sclerosis, 122, 165
mystery, 43
myths, 39, 45, 136, 138, 155

National Skills Academy, 13
natural rights, 78-80
nature, 78, 95, 96
Nazism, 138
New Zealand, 36
news-media, 80-6, 100, 101
Newton, Isaac, 142
NHS, 1-14, 30, 102-3, 108, 109, 113-14
NHS Constitution
  access to services, 6
  accountability, 7

NHS Constitution *cont.*
  clinical negligence, 6
  definition of health, 102, 113
  patient goals, 169
  Principle 1, 1–2
  Principle 4, 3, 5
  values-based recruitment (VBR), 12, 21
NHS Litigation Authority, 6
Nicholson, Jack, 40
nicotine, 155
Night of Broken Glass, 138
Nightingale, Florence, 41
non-compliance, 153, 180, 181
non-maleficence, 126–27
Northern Territory Intervntion, 79
nursing, 7–9, 41, 90

Obama, Barack, 140
oceanographers, 151
Once Flew Over a Cuckoo's Nest, 40
open mindfulness, 148–52
opportunity costs, 91
organic farming, 98–9
Orwell, George, 83, 134–35

painting, 52
paternalism, 174–75
patient advocacy, 172
patients, 55, 57–8
payment, for treatment, 6
people with disabilities, 77–8
persisting ethics, 120-21, 124, 128, 153
Peutherer, Vanessa, 4–5, 11, 61, 70, 175–76, 180
Pfeiffer, Dr Ehrenfried, 98–99
pharmaceutical products, 7
phenomenon teaching, 74
plant pot, 41
plants, 94–99
plastics, 44
pneumonia, 59
Posner, Eric, 79
Postman, Neil, 82–83
poverty, 91, 138
Power, Michael, 69
preferences, 25–6, 28, 31, 60
Price, Alan, 27
Principles of Biomedical Ethics, 126
private health care, 6
problems, 45–47
The Problems of Philosophy, 50–51
Proctor, Reuben, 117
progress, 89, 90, 93
propaganda, 73, 132, 156–58
psychiatrists, 153
public health, 154
purpose, 101

racial discrimination, 59
rain forests, 33
reality, 37–46, 47, 117
Rebels Against the Future, 67
reform, 17–18
religion, 82, 97, 98
respect for autonomy, 92–3
respect for others, 12, 13, 16, 76
right to know, 19–20, 43
rights, 58–9, 72–3, 101
risk, 49–53, 60, 64, 72, 75, 107, 123, 127, 130
Roach, Simone, 6–7
road traffic accidents, 52
Robinson, Ken, 55
Ronaldo, 58
rugby, 115
Russell, Bertrand, 37–9, 40, 95, 96, 97, 102, 117

Sagan, Carl, 89
Sale, Kirkpatrick, 91–2
schizophrenia, 40, 108
schools, 18–19, 99–100
The Secret Life of Plants, 96–97, 99
Seedhouse, Charles Donald, 122–24
Selak, Frano, 74–5, 76
self-management, 174
separateness, 42–5, 47, 49, 103, 108, 109, 127, 162, 171–79, 182
scepticism, 141
smoking, 5, 41, 48, 61–62, 154–58
strikes, 115
suicide, 110, 116, 120, 170
Suli, 74
Sun, 85
superbugs, 7
symbols, 36–8
systemic change, 171–72

tardive dyskinesia, 7
targets, 12
teaching, 573
technology, 88, 130,
TED stockings, 130–1
telecommunications, 44
telegraph, 84
television, 82
texture, 52
Think Screen, 168
Thomsen, Lars, 117
thromboembolism-deterrent (TED) hoses, 180–81
Tide: The Science and Lore of the Greatest Force on Earth, 150–52
Tompkins, Peter, 96, 98
Twitter, 84

Universit73s, 55

values
    Army, 31
    British Army, 16–17
    Coca Cola Company, 14–15
    delusion, 59–60, 64
    hierarchies, 28
    as labels, 23, 28, 29, 64
    McDonalds, 15–16, 31
    nature of, 24–8
    NHS, 1–14, 31
    official view, 1–7, 21–22, 35, 60
    and ourselves, 60–62
    and reform, 23–24
    schools, 18–20
    value judgements, 143
    values statements, 1, 3, 5, 7, 15–19, 22
Values Exchange, 10, 60, 140, 168

values-based recruitment (VBR), 13–14, 20–1, 24–25, 31, 152, 171
Vanderbilt, Tom, 131
Veganissimo A to Z, 117
vegetarians, 116, 134
Victorial Hospital, 41
violence, 137
Vize, Richard, 24
Voltaire, 137

Walmart, 16
weapons, 95, 139
weeds, 95
wheat, 94–5
windows, 41

Yamagochi, Tsutomu, 75